THE KEGEL FIX

RECHARGING FEMALE PELVIC, SEXUAL AND URINARY HEALTH

THE KEGEL FIX

RECHARGING FEMALE PELVIC, SEXUAL AND URINARY HEALTH

ANDREW L. SIEGEL, M.D.

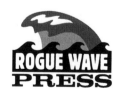

ROGUE WAVE PRESS

Published by ROGUE WAVE PRESS

Copyright © 2016 by Andrew L. Siegel, M.D.

Printed in the United States of America

First printing 2016

ISBN: 978-0-9830617-5-5

To order additional copies of this book: www.TheKegelFix.com

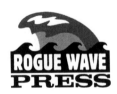

I dedicate this book with much love to my father, Jerald Siegel, a retired urologist who is 85 years young and going strong. I have the greatest respect and admiration for him not only for being my dad (and a fantastic grandfather), but also for being a skilled physician and surgeon who had a pivotal influence on my entering the field of urology.

It was a pleasure and honor to work hand in hand with him for well over a decade. It presented tremendous opportunities, although treading the fine line between our personal and professional lives was at times challenging. For example, I was always perplexed about how to address him in the operating room as we performed surgery together: "Dr. Siegel" too formal . . . "Jerry" too casual . . . "Dad" too child-like. Regardless, he has always been an inspiring role model, especially because of his integrity, compassion and humility. I frequently see his former patients who send him their regards, often referring to him as "salt of the earth."

Thank you again for paying for my education and I am genuinely sorry that our urology legacy stops with my generation!

TABLE OF CONTENTS

ACKNOWLEDGMENTS

A heartfelt thanks, as always, to Les, my faithful partner, steadfast help-mate, collaborator, confidante, editor, tandem bike mate and best friend. She has always been an unwavering advocate who has provided me with unconditional support, never begrudging me the substantial amounts of time I have spent pursuing my passions. She has been a source of clarity, solace and sustenance and a loving and stalwart fixture in my existence in a world too often marked by randomness, chaos and lunacy. Her years of experience in the publishing field as an editor at Prentice Hall and director of publicity and promotion at Random House prior to becoming a mom and CEO of our household have been of great benefit in terms of converting my rambling into coherent prose and medical mumbo-jumbo into readable English. In addition to her editing assistance, she provided invaluable input regarding the title and cover. For all of this, and so much more, I am forever grateful.

My great appreciation to Professor Grace Dorey, one of the world's leading experts in the field of pelvic floor physiotherapy and Emeritus Professor of Physiotherapy/Urology at the University of the West of England, Bristol and Consultant Physiotherapist at The Nuffield Hospital, Tauton, England. In addition to reviewing the manuscript, she was gracious enough to write the foreword.

A tremendous debt of gratitude to Jeff Siegel for his assistance with all things technical: cover, e-book, website and book trailer. Creative kudos to Ashley Halsey for her medical illustrations.

I am indebted and beholden to the innovative and pioneering work of internationally-recognized gynecologist Dr. Arnold Kegel, who popularized female pelvic floor exercises in the 1940s and whose legacy bears his name—"Kegel" exercises.

Finally, a special thanks to my patients, who have entrusted me with their urological care. They have opened up their lives and hearts, have shared personal and intimate details and have been among my most important and informative teachers, providing me with a wealth of knowledge not to be found in medical textbooks or journals. Without them, this book would not have been possible.

FOREWORD

Dr Andrew Siegel has done it again! After producing his highly successful and unique book for men titled: Male Pelvic Fitness: Optimizing Sexual and Urinary Health, he is to be congratulated for now writing a brilliant book for women titled: *The Kegel Fix: Recharging Female Pelvic, Sexual and Urinary Health*.

It is unusual for a top urologist to be interested in conservative therapy to this extent and to champion the use of pelvic floor exercises. He has explored the subject thoroughly and has produced an outstanding book containing detailed information of benefit to medical professionals and their patients. Indeed, it will be of value to all women from adolescence onwards.

Over the past 60 years, physical therapists have been teaching pelvic floor exercises to women suffering from the embarrassment and often devastation of urinary leakage and sometimes faecal incontinence after childbirth. Now we know that pelvic floor training should be part of every woman's fitness programme in order to prevent the onset of a plethora of pelvic problems.

In a clear, logical and scientific approach, Dr. Siegel has researched the mechanics of the female pelvic floor and has shown readers how, with the right regimen of exercises, urinary incontinence can be avoided, treated and, importantly, prevented from returning.

There is a concise chapter on pelvic pain illuminating the importance of pelvic floor muscle relaxation in order to relieve the awful aching that muscle spasm can produce in this delicate area.

Uniquely, Dr Siegel explores in depth the role of pelvic floor training for a range of sexual dysfunction in order for women (and their partners) to have sexual fulfillment as a major part of their relationship.

Importantly, there are two chapters detailing firstly active then resisted pelvic floor training, which cover a range of available resistance devices.

It is my wish that this excellent book will be made available in all English-speaking countries and translated into other languages so that all women (and their partners) can enjoy richer and fuller lives.

Professor Grace Dorey MBE, FCSP, PhD
Consultant Physiotherapist
Devon, UK
www.yourpelvicfloor.co.uk

COMMON ABBREVIATIONS

BC	bulbocavernosus muscle
BCR	bulbo-cavernosus reflex
DIY	do it yourself
IC	ischiocavernosus muscle
OAB	overactive bladder
PC	pubococcygeus muscle
PFM	pelvic floor muscle
PFMT	pelvic floor muscle training
POP	pelvic organ prolapse
PT	physical therapy
SUI	stress urinary incontinence
UUI	urgency urinary incontinence

PREFACE

The pelvic floor muscles (PFM) have long been recognized as vital for supporting the pelvic organs, for healthy sexual function and for ensuring urinary and bowel control. Additionally, the PFM contribute to core muscle stability and provide postural support. The PFM not only anatomically and functionally link the pelvic organs—the vagina, uterus, bladder and rectum—but also affect the independent function of each.

Exercises of the PFM are not a new concept, dating back over 6000 years ago to Chinese Taoism. The Yogis of ancient India practiced similar exercises, assuming the proper posture and performing rhythmic contractions of the anal sphincter (considered to be one of the superficial PFM). Hippocrates and Galen described PFM exercises in ancient Greece and Rome, respectively, where they were performed in the baths and gymnasiums and were thought to promote longevity as well as general health, sexual health and spiritual health.

For centuries thereafter, however, PFM exercises were thrust into the "dark." Fast-forward to the 1930s when Margaret Morris, a British physical therapist, described PFM exercises as a means of preventing and treating urinary and bowel control issues. Then came the 1940s, when the seminal work of Dr. Arnold Kegel resulted in PFM exercises achieving the stature and acclaim that they deserved. Kegel's legacy is the actual name that many use to refer to PFM exercises—"Kegels" or "Kegel exercises." Kegel determined that a successful PFM program must include muscle education, feedback, resistance, and progressive intensity. He stressed the need for pelvic floor muscle *training* (PFMT) as opposed to casual *exercises*, emphasizing the importance of a diligently performed and dedicated routine.

Despite Kegel's PFMT regimen proving effective for many female pelvic problems—including those of pelvic support, sexual function and urinary/bowel control—what is currently referred to as Kegel exercises bears little resemblance to what Kegel so brilliantly described in his classic series of medical articles sixty-five years ago. His PFMT regimen incorporated a critical focus and intensity that are unfortunately not upheld in most of today's programs.

Sadly, easy-to-follow pelvic exercise programs or well-designed means of enabling PFMT are lacking. In the post-Kegel era, we have regressed to the Dark Ages with respect to PFMT. Today's programs typically involve vague verbal instructions and perhaps a pamphlet suggesting a several month regimen of ten or so PFM contractions squeezing against no resistance, to be done several times daily during "down" times. These programs are typically static and do not offer more challenging exercises over time. Such Kegel "knockoffs" and watered-down, adulterated versions—even those publicized by esteemed medical institutions—lack in guidance, feedback and rigor, demand little time and effort and often ignore the benefit of resistance, thus accounting for their ineffectiveness. With women often unable to identify their PFM or properly perform the training, outcomes are less than favorable and the frustration level and high abandonment rate with these PFMT regimens are hardly surprising. Thus, PFMT remains an often ignored, neglected, misunderstood, under-respected and under-exploited resource.

The Challenge of Pelvic Floor Muscle Training (PFMT)

There are several obstacles to implementing PFMT: the PFM themselves, physicians who might try to take on administering the training, and patients.

The first challenge is that it is not an easy task to motivate people to exercise muscles that are not visible. Moreover, because the PFM are hidden muscles that are most often used subconsciously, teaching *conscious* engagement of them in order to develop muscle memory is difficult.

Secondly, many physicians have received little or no training on pelvic floor issues and those that have hardly have the time to adequately teach PFMT. Furthermore, most medical doctors are not particularly interested in this task, which can be burdensome, time-consuming and not reimbursed by medical insurance. The bottom line is do not expect to learn much about Kegels from your doctor.

Thirdly, patients—most of whom know nothing about these mysterious muscles—must be educated on the specifics of the PFM, the proper techniques of conditioning them and the practical application of the exercises to their specific issues. In our instant gratification world, many patients are not motivated or enthused about slow fixes and the investment of time and effort required of an exercise program—which lacks the sizzle and quick fix of pharmaceuticals or the operating room—so patient compliance and willingness to pursue the exercises are important and oftentimes limiting factors. Additionally, many women with pelvic issues are reluctant to seek help for a variety of reasons. These include embarrassment about the very personal nature of their problems, the misconception that their pelvic troubles are always an expected consequence of pregnancy or aging, a lack of awareness that help is available and the fear that surgery will be the only treatment option.

WHO KNEW? *Many of my patients have "tried" PFM exercises without noting improvement. When I ask them to squeeze their PFM during a pelvic exam, they often contract the wrong muscles, usually the abdominals, buttocks or thigh muscles. Others bear down as if they are moving their bowels, instead of doing just the opposite—drawing up and in. Some lift their hips into the air, a good core exercise but not one that isolates and fully engages the PFM. Others cannot do a PFM contraction at all.*

For years I managed these stumbling blocks by explaining PFM exercises as best as I could and handing patients written materials. I found this to be inadequate and ineffective, so I created a YouTube video to be used as a supplement to my office instruction and handout. Although more a general source of information about the PFM rather than a specific training regimen, this video was well received by my patients and many others, with hundreds of thousands of views to date. Its popularity informed me of the vital need and unmet demand for an effective means by which PFMT could be made easily accessible.

WHO KNEW? *With respect to PFMT, most medical practices give patients only verbal instructions or nothing at all. In more ideal circumstances, patients receive a leaflet, but that is as far as it typically goes.*

So, if one is so motivated to learn about their PFM and how to exercise them, how does one obtain information? Many navigate the Internet as a go-to source of enlightenment. However, the content on the Internet is poorly regulated, unfiltered, and is often lacking in quality, substantiated information. Many of the websites devoted to PFMT are promotional in nature. Most of the online PFMT guidance is far too basic and incomplete.

Additionally, there are a number of PFM applications (apps) available for download. Many are follow-along tutorials that provide a timer for doing PFM exercises and audio and visual cues for contracting and relaxing the PFM. Regrettably, they all have a bare minimum of in-depth content, medical focus and meaningful instruction, serving mainly as timing prompters. None provide the foundational knowledge upon which PFMT is based. The bottom line is that quality resources to improve pelvic floor health are sorely lacking in availability.

Physicians who want their patients to pursue PFMT but do not have the time nor the interest to teach them may consider referring them for pelvic floor physical therapy (PT). Physical therapists who specialize in pelvic floor issues deal with a wide range of pelvic floor dysfunctions ranging from PFM weakness to PFM tension (a condition in which the PFM are over-contracted, causing pelvic pain and sexual, urinary and bowel problems). Pelvic floor PT sessions can be a lifesaver for women who are incapable of mastering PFMT. There is compelling evidence that women do better with supervised PFMT regimens than they do without. I liken the pelvic floor physical therapist to a "personal trainer" for the PFM. The downside of PT is that it is time-consuming and expensive, with variable coverage depending upon the insurance carrier.

WHO KNEW? *In France, the government subsidizes the cost of PFMT after childbirth ("La rééducation périnéale après accouchement"). It includes up to 20 sessions of pelvic PT intended to firm and tone the postnatal PFM and "re-educate" the vagina. This program has been successful on an individual and national basis, as new mothers are thrilled to have pelvic health professionals at their disposal and France boasts the second highest birth rate in the European Union. A coincidence? . . . I think not!*

WHO KNEW? *Seattle-based Herman & Wallace Pelvic Rehabilitation Institute (HermanWallace.com), founded by experts in pelvic floor dysfunction Hollis Herman and Kathe Wallace, has a practitioner directory of USA pelvic floor physiotherapists.*

Many women are interested in pursuing PFMT, not necessarily under the guidance of a health professional such as a PT or MD, but more as part of an "exercise" routine as opposed to a "medical" program. What about "Do It Yourself" (DIY) programs? The first problem with DIY is in finding the proper plan and the second problem is seeing it through to reap meaningful results. The majority of those who try DIY Kegels cannot find a program that provides the foundational background and the means of isolating and exercising the PFM in a progressively more challenging fashion. It is the equivalent of giving someone a set of weights and expecting them to engage in a weight training program without the essential knowledge and principles of anatomy and function, a specific exercise routine and the supervision to go along with the equipment— which would most certainly doom them to failure.

This leads me to the purposes and objectives I have in writing this book. The consequences of weakened PFM are urinary and bowel control problems, dropped pelvic organs and sexual dysfunction, taboo issues that many women do not have much knowledge about nor consider topics appropriate for conversation. I wish to explore these "off-limit" subjects that are the final frontier of uncharted territory in women's health. As the word *doctor* derives from the Latin *docere* ("to teach"), my intention is to engage and educate readers in order that they achieve pelvic health literacy, including an understanding of the pelvic consequences of pregnancy, labor, childbirth, menopause and lifestyle. My goal is to enhance the quality of life of women by showing them how to tap into the powers of their PFM and how to "snap, clench and squeeze" their way to a healthy, fit, firm and toned vagina and PFM. I aim to demystify the PFM—out of sight, out of mind, and often misunderstood—and make PFMT less intimidating and more accessible.

My ambition is to help deliver PFMT from the Dark Ages and contribute to the "pelvic revolution," restoring PFMT to the classic sense established by Arnold Kegel—a "renaissance" to a new era of "pelvic enlightenment." I introduce new age, next generation Kegels—progressive, home-based, tailored exercise programs consisting of strength and endurance training regimens that are designed and customized for the specific pelvic floor dysfunction at hand. My intent is to provide the means for women to master pelvic fitness and optimize pelvic support and sexual, urinary and bowel function, thereby empowering them from within.

Finally, because many women who are taught PFMT do not understand how to put their newfound knowledge and skills to real life use, my ultimate desire is to teach *functional pelvic fitness*—practical and actionable means of applying PFM proficiency to daily tasks and common everyday activities. There is no better time than the present to begin PFMT in order to prevent, delay or treat pelvic floor dysfunction, beneficial from bedroom to bathroom.

Be Well.

Dr. Andrew Siegel

1   PELVIC FLOOR MUSCLES (PFM) 101

This chapter provides basic information on the pelvic floor muscles that is essential for understanding the chapters that follow.

WHO KNEW?   *Everything sounds better in French. Which sounds sexier, "pelvic floor" muscles or "Bellefleur" muscles? I often use Siri to dictate my thoughts on my Apple iPhone, and when I say "pelvic floor muscles"—probably a little too fast—Siri interprets it as "Bellefleur" muscles. Bellefleur happens to be the French term for "beautiful flower," an apt description of the female PFM. This is a "Siriously" fortuitous mistake!*

What Are the Kegel Muscles? Where Are They? What Do They Do?

The pelvic floor muscles (PFM), commonly known as the "Kegel muscles," are a hammock of muscles that form the underside of the pelvis. They are also referred to as the "saddle" muscles, because you sit on them when you are seated on a bicycle. They are part of the "core" muscles, which are the "barrel" of muscles comprising the torso, consisting of the abdominal muscles in front, the lumbar muscles in back, the diaphragm muscle forming the roof and the PFM forming the floor. The core muscles are responsible for stabilizing the pelvis and holding the spine erect.

The *deep* PFM (*pubococcygeus, iliococcygeus, coccygeus*) span from

Figure 1. Core Muscles

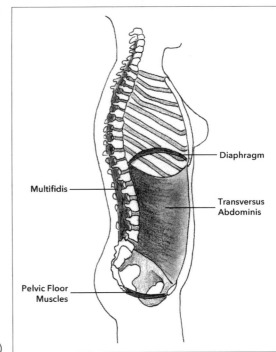

Diaphragm

Multifidis

Transversus
Abdominis

Pelvic Floor
Muscles

Figure 2. Deep PFM
(Abdominal View)

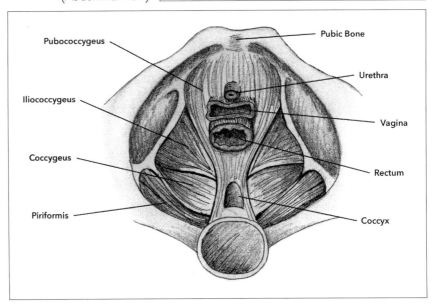

Pubococcygeus

Pubic Bone

Urethra

Iliococcygeus

Vagina

Coccygeus

Rectum

Piriformis

Coccyx

the pubic bone in front to the tailbone in the back, and from pelvic sidewall to pelvic sidewall, between the "sit" bones.

The *superficial* PFM (*ischiocavernosus, bulbocavernosus, transverse perineal, anal sphincter*) are situated under the surface of the external genitals and anus.

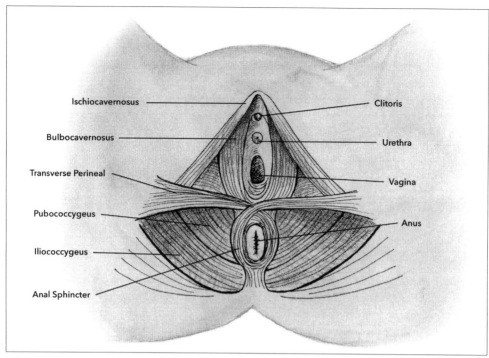

Figure 3. Superficial and Deep PFM (Vaginal View)

The PFM muscles are intertwined with the muscles of the vagina, bladder and rectum. These muscles provide support for the pelvic organs, contribute to the control mechanism of the urinary and intestinal tracts and play a vital role in sexual function.

WHO KNEW?   *Many women are unaware of their PFM and are unable to identify them, have no notion as to how to squeeze them nor know that this is even something that they should be doing.*

What Is the Problem and What Is the Fix?

One of every four women in the USA has symptoms due to weakened PFM and many more have pelvic floor weakness that is not yet symptomatic. Many others have symptoms from PFM that are too tense. More than 10% of American women will undergo surgery for pelvic floor issues—commonly for stress urinary incontinence (urinary leakage with coughing, sneezing and/or exercise) and pelvic organ prolapse (sagging of one or more of the pelvic organs into the vaginal canal and at times outside the vaginal opening)—with up to 30% requiring repeat surgical procedures.

As a urologist who cares for many female patients, my office hour sessions bear witness to common complaints that are due to a variety of pelvic floor problems:

"Every time I go on the trampoline with my daughter, my bladder leaks. The same thing happens when I jump rope with her."
—Brittany, age 29

"My vagina is just not the same as it was before I had my kids. It's loose to the extent that I can't keep a tampon in."   —Allyson, age 38

"As soon as I get near my home, I get a tremendous urge to empty my bladder. I have to scramble to find my keys and can't seem to put the key in the door fast enough. I make a beeline to the bathroom, but often have an accident on the way."   —Jan, age 57

"Sex is so different now. I don't get easily aroused the way I did when I was younger. Intercourse doesn't feel like it used to and I don't climax as often or as intensively as I did before having my three children. My husband now seems to get 'lost' in my vagina. I worry about satisfying him."   —Leah, age 43

"When I bent over to pick up my granddaughter, I felt a strange sensation between my legs, as if something gave way. I rushed to the bathroom and used a hand mirror and saw a bulge coming out of my vagina. It looked like a pink ball and I felt like all my insides were falling out."   —Karen, age 66

"I have been experiencing on and off stabbing pain in my lower abdomen, groin and vagina. It is worse after urinating and moving my bowels. Sex is usually impossible because of how much it hurts."
—Tara, age 31

These issues come under the broad term *pelvic floor dysfunction*, a common condition causing symptoms that can range from mildly annoying to debilitating. Pelvic floor dysfunction develops when the PFM are traumatized, injured or neglected. Pelvic floor muscle training (PFMT), a.k.a. "Kegels," has the capacity for improving all of these situations.

PFM fitness is critical to healthy pelvic function and is an important element of overall health and fitness. PFMT is a safe, natural, non-invasive, first-line self-improvement approach to pelvic floor dysfunction that should be considered before more aggressive, more costly and riskier treatments. We engage in exercise programs for virtually every other muscle group in the body and should not ignore the PFM, which when trained can become toned and robust, capable of supporting and sustaining pelvic anatomy and function to the maximum. Should one fail to benefit from such conservative management, more aggressive options always remain available.

PFMT can be beneficial for the following categories of pelvic floor dysfunction: *weakened pelvic support* (descent and sagging of the pelvic organs including the bladder, urethra, uterus, rectum and vagina itself); *vaginal laxity* (looseness); *altered sexual* and *orgasmic function*; *stress urinary incontinence* (urinary leakage with coughing and exertion); *overactive bladder* (the sudden urge to urinate with leakage often occurring before being able to get to the bathroom); *pelvic pain due to PFM spasm*; and *bowel urgency* and *incontinence*. Additionally, PFMT improves core strength, lumbar stability and spinal alignment, aids in preventing back pain and helps prepare one for pregnancy, labor and delivery. PFMT can be advantageous not only for those with any of the previously mentioned problems, but also as a means of helping to prevent them in the first place. Exercising the PFM in your 20s and 30s can help avert problems in your 40s, 50s, 60s and beyond.

Who Knew? There are numerous benefits to increasing the strength, tone and endurance of your PFM. Even if you approach PFMT with one specific functional goal in mind, all domains will benefit, a nice advantage of conditioning such a versatile group of muscles.

Why Bother Exercising Your PFM?

The PFM are out of sight and out of mind; however, they have important functions, so are muscles that you should be exercising. PFMT is based upon solid exercise science and can help maintain PFM integrity and optimal function into old age. The PFM are "plastic" and capable of making adaptive changes when targeted exercise is applied to them. Their structure and function can be enhanced, resulting in broader, thicker and firmer PFM with a stronger resting tone and the ability to generate a powerful contraction at will. PFMT can be effective in stabilizing, relieving, improving and even preventing issues with pelvic support, sexual function, and urinary and bowel control. In addition to the muscle-training benefit of PFMT, it also supports tissue healing by stimulating the flow of oxygenated, nutritionally rich blood to the vagina and other pelvic organs.

Because of pregnancy, labor and delivery, the PFM get stretched more than any other muscle group in the body. Through PFMT, the PFM have the capacity of rebounding from this obstetrical "trauma," recovering tone and function. Prenatal PFMT can help fortify the PFM in preparation for pregnancy, labor and delivery. PFMT involves gaining facility with both the contracting and the relaxing phases of PFM function. One might think erroneously that PFMT could lead to a more difficult birth because of stronger and tighter PFM; however, PFMT also facilitates better *relaxation* of the PFM that can ease the childbirth process.

WHO KNEW? *Tail wagging in dogs is the responsibility of the PFM. Weak PFM are rarely observed in such animals—despite giving birth to large litters—suggesting that with constant movement of the tail the PFM are exercised sufficiently to maintain tone or to restore function following injury.*

WHO KNEW? *The distinction between well-toned and flabby PFM is similar to the difference between well toned as opposed to flabby leg muscles, although not so readily apparent since the PFM are internal muscles.*

What Exactly Is PFM Dysfunction and What Causes It?

PFM "dysfunction" is a common condition referring to when the PFM are not functioning properly. PFM dysfunction ranges from "low tone" to "high tone." Low tone occurs when the PFM lack in strength and endurance and is often associated with stress urinary incontinence, pelvic organ prolapse and altered sexual function. High tone occurs when the PFM are too tense and unable to relax, giving rise to a pain syndrome known as tension myalgia.

The PFM can become weakened, flabby and poorly functional with pregnancy, labor, childbirth, menopause, weight gain, a sedentary lifestyle, poor posture, sports injuries, pelvic trauma, chronic straining, pelvic surgery, diabetes, tobacco use, steroid use, and disuse atrophy (not exercising the PFM). Sexual inactivity can lead to their loss of tone, texture and function. With aging there is a decline in the bulk and contractility of the PFM, often resulting in PFM dysfunction.

WHO KNEW? *PFM dysfunction often causes symptoms in several domains, e.g., women with urinary incontinence often have trouble achieving orgasm, both problems contributed to by weakened PFM.*

WHO KNEW?   *Poor posture—a common occurrence in women suffering with osteoporosis who often develop compression fractures that cause them to slump—can be an important factor in causing urinary incontinence and other pelvic floor issues because of postural-related altered pressures on the pelvic floor. PFMT can significantly reduce incontinence episodes.*

WHO KNEW?   *"Cyclist's Vulva." Chronic compression of the genitals against the bicycle seat from prolonged time in the saddle can traumatize the genital blood vessels, nerves and PFM. This can result in decreased genital sensation and sexual dysfunction.*

Why Are the PFM So Vital to Your Health?

The PFM are perhaps the most versatile yet under-appreciated muscle group in your body. They provide vaginal tone, support to the pelvic organs, a healthy sexual response—enhancing arousal and orgasm— and urinary and bowel sphincter control. They play a key role in your ability to carry and deliver a baby as well as contributing to the mobility and stability of your torso.

WHO KNEW?   *A simplified way of thinking of the female pelvic organs—bladder, uterus and bowel—is as "storage containers" for urine, fetuses, and stool, respectively. Each organ is connected to the outside world by tubular structures, the urethra, vagina and anal canal, respectively, through which flow the contents of the organs. The PFM play a strong role in compressing the tubes for storage and relaxing them for emptying.*

WHO KNEW?   *The PFM may literally be at the bottom of the barrel of our core muscles, but in terms of their important functions, they are figuratively furthermost from the "bottom of the barrel."*

Why Are the PFM So Mysterious?

Strong puritanical roots in our culture influence our thoughts and feelings about our nether regions; as a result, they often fail to command the respect and attention that other areas of our bodies do. Frequently ignored and/or neglected, this area of the body rarely sees the light of day and most women never think about exercising the important functional muscles in this sector of their anatomy. Most of us can probably point out our "bi's" (biceps), "tri's" (triceps), "quads" (quadriceps), "pecs" (pectorals), etc., but who really knows *where* their "pelvs" (PFM) are located? For that matter, who even knows *what* they are and *how* they contribute to pelvic health? Your leg muscles might look sexy and lean and provide you with the ability to walk, but think for a moment about the PFM. How essential—yet taken for granted—is sphincter control, support of our pelvic organs and, of course, their key contribution to sexual function?

Unlike the glitzy, for show, external, mirror-appealing glamour muscles, the PFM are humble muscles that are shrouded in secrecy, hidden from view, unseen and behind the scenes, often unrecognized and misunderstood. The PFM mystique is contributed to by their mysterious powers, which straddle the gamut of being vital for what may be considered the most pleasurable and sublime of human pursuits—sex—but equally integral to what may be considered the least refined of human activities—bowel and bladder function.

WHO KNEW?   *You can't see your PFM in the mirror. Because they are out of sight and out of mind, they are often neglected, but there is great merit in exercising important hidden muscles, including the heart, diaphragm and PFM. Although the PFM are not muscles of "glamour," they are the muscles of "amour," fundamental to sexual function.*

What Is the Muscle Function of the PFM?

Whereas most skeletal muscles function as *movers* (joint movement and locomotion), the PFM are unique in that they function as *stabilizers*—helping to keep the pelvic organs in proper position—and *compressors*—helping to tighten the vagina, urethra and rectum—important to urinary and bowel control as well as to sexual function. During sex the PFM activate, causing a surge of genital blood flow that helps lubrication and clitoral engorgement; at the time of orgasm, the PFM contract rhythmically.

WHO KNEW?   *Without functioning PFM, your organs would dangle out of your pelvis, you would be wearing adult diapers and your sexual function would be nil.*

What Happens to the PFM With Childbirth?

PFM take a beating from pregnancy, labor and vaginal delivery. Pregnancy incurs maternal weight gain, a change in body posture, pregnancy-related hormonal changes and the pressure of a growing uterus and fetal weight, all of which may reduce the supportive and sphincter (urinary and bowel control) functions of the PFM.

Labor is called so for a genuine reason! The hours you spend pushing and straining are often very unkind to the PFM. *Elective* Caesarian section avoids labor and affords protection to the PFM, but prolonged labor that results in an *emergency* C-section is equally as potentially damaging to the PFM as vaginal delivery.

Vaginal delivery is the ultimate traumatic event to the PFM. The soft tissues of the pelvis (including PFM) get crushed in the "vise" between your baby's bony skull and your own bony pelvis and are simply no match for the hardness and inflexibility of these bones. The PFM and connective tissues are frequently stretched, if not torn, from their attachments to the pubic bone and pelvic sidewalls, and the nerves to the pelvic floor are often affected as well. The undesirable consequences of obstetric "trauma" include altered PFM anatomy with loss of vaginal tone and function, a.k.a. birth-related laxity (looseness).

Studies measuring PFM strength before and after first delivery show a decrease in PFM strength in about 50% of women. Vaginal delivery is much more likely to reduce PFM strength than delivery via C-section. Not surprisingly, following delivery, the larger the measured diameter of the vaginal opening, the weaker the vaginal strength.

WHO KNEW? *After a vaginal delivery, things "down there" are often just not quite the same. The vagina beomes looser and more open, the vaginal lining becomes dryer and hormonal-related pigmentation changes often cause a darker appearance of the vulva.*

WHO KNEW? *The most extreme form of birth trauma is obstetric fistula, a not uncommon, horrific problem often occurring in poverty-stricken countries where pregnant women have poor access to obstetric care. It happens after enduring days of "obstructed" labor, with the baby's head persistently pushing against the mother's pelvic bones during contractions. This prevents pelvic blood flow and causes tissue death, resulting in a hole called a "fistula" between the vagina and the bladder and/or vagina and rectum. When birth finally occurs, the baby is often stillborn. The long-term consequences for the mother are severe urinary and bowel incontinence, shame and social isolation.*

2 TEN REASONS TO EXERCISE YOUR PFM

1. To enable you to have a more comfortable pregnancy, a smoother labor and delivery, and a faster recovery.

2. To improve/prevent pelvic relaxation (dropped bladder, uterus, rectum, etc.) and vaginal laxity (looseness).

3. To improve/prevent sexual and orgasmic issues.

4. To enhance sexual pleasure for you and your partner.

5. To improve/prevent stress urinary incontinence (leakage with coughing, sneezing, exercise, etc.).

6. To improve/prevent urinary and bowel urgency ("gotta go") and urgency urinary and bowel incontinence ("gotta go" and can't make it to the bathroom on time to prevent an accident).

7. To improve/prevent pelvic pain due to pelvic tension myalgia by learning how to properly relax the PFM.

8. To help prevent pelvic impairments from high impact sports and saddle sports (e.g., cycling, motorcycling and horseback riding).

9. To improve core strength, posture, lumbar stability, alignment and balance.

10. To maintain good health and youthful vitality.

3

ARNOLD KEGEL

Dr. Arnold Kegel (1894-1981) was a gynecologist who taught at the University of Southern California School of Medicine. In the late 1940s, he was singularly responsible for popularizing female pelvic floor muscle exercises in order to improve sexual and urinary health. (It is important to know that although these exercises were designed particularly for women after childbirth, they are equally and successfully applicable to the broader population of women.)

Kegel used the principle of *functional restoration* of an isolated group of muscles—already well established in orthopedics, plastic surgery and physical medicine and rehabilitation—applying it to the PFM. His legacy is the pelvic floor exercises that bear his name, known as "Kegel exercises." He invented a device called the *perineometer* that was placed in the vagina to create resistance and to measure the strength of PFM contractions, thus providing biofeedback.

Kegel described PFM exercise as an effort to "draw in" the perineum, the tissues between the vagina and anus. Kegel's goal was for "broader, thicker and firmer" PFM and a tighter muscular plane through which the urethra, vagina and rectum pass.

Arnold Kegel did not invent pelvic floor exercises, but popularized them in women. Recall that PFM exercises have actually been around for thousands of years. Kegel came onto the scene in the 1940s and made the link between childbirth and PFM dysfunction resulting in stress urinary incontinence, pelvic laxity and impaired sexual function.

Kegel observed that in women before childbirth the vaginal canal was typically tight, firm and closed to a high level, offering resistance to the examining finger in every direction. Oftentimes after delivery the vaginal canal became looser and flabbier, offering little resistance to the examining finger. Kegel questioned his patients about their sexual function after childbirth, concluding that sex felt different after delivery and that sexuality was closely related to vaginal muscle tone and was capable of being improved with proper exercises. Additionally, Kegel observed that about one in three new mothers suffered with stress urinary incontinence.

WHO KNEW? *In one of Kegel's classic articles, he referred to a tribe of natives in Africa whose pelvic anatomy was observed to be unusually firm and intact. This was thought to be due to exercises of the vaginal muscles contracted upon the distended fingers of midwives starting several days after birth.*

According to Kegel, the reasons for pursuing PFMT are the following: vaginal looseness; weakened, poorly toned or poorly functional PFM; pelvic organ bulging and prolapse; stress urinary incontinence; impaired sexual function; and "pelvic fatigue" (a rather vague symptom). He discovered that with his regimen, a vagina initially admitting three fingers could be tightened to a snug, well-closed vagina admitting only one finger, with the results sustained over time.

WHO KNEW? *One of Kegel's aims was to improve vaginal muscle tone so that a contraceptive diaphragm could be held in place without falling out.*

Kegel wrote: "*Muscles that have lost tone, texture and function can be restored to use by active exercise against progressive resistance since muscles increase in strength in direct proportion to the demands placed upon them.*" He believed that a minimum of twenty hours of exercise would be necessary to obtain maximal development of the PFM.

Dr. Kegel wrote a number of classic articles including: *The Non-Surgical Treatment of Genital Relaxation*; *Progressive Resistance Exercise in the Functional Restoration of the Perineal Muscles*; *Sexual Functions of the Pubococcygeus Muscle*; and *The Physiologic Treatment of Poor Tone and Function of the Genital Muscles and of Urinary Stress Incontinence*. Their content is summarized in the paragraphs that follow.

Since pregnancy, labor and delivery invariably inflict damage to pelvic anatomy—often resulting in flabby, weakened and poorly functional PFM—Kegel designed a PFMT program that he used successfully on thousands of his patients. His objectives were a tighter, toned and firmer vaginal canal with improved urinary control, pelvic support and sexuality.

WHO KNEW? *Kegel observed that the tricky thing about PFM injuries as opposed to injuries of external muscles is that the PFM are internal, hidden muscles that cannot be directly observed and thus their injuries are* *masked.*

His program of PFM rehabilitation incorporated four important principles. The first was that of *muscle education*—an understanding of PFM anatomy and function. This enabled muscle memory—the development of the nerve pathway from the brain to the PFM. The second principle was *feedback* to confirm to the exerciser that the proper muscles were being used, important since studies have shown that up to 50% of women who think they are doing PFM exercises properly are actually squeezing other muscles, typically the rectus (abs), gluteal (butt) and adductor (thigh) muscles. Feedback served as a means of demonstrating that initial weak and irregular contractions became strong and sustained and a way of measuring and monitoring progress over time as PFM strength increased. The feedback also provided motivation; by demonstrating improvement over time, the exerciser was incentivized and inspired to keep at the program. The third principle was *resistance*, which further challenged the PFM to work harder to increase their tone, texture and bulk. Resistance was capable of rapidly escalating PFM strength and endurance since the growth of muscles occurs in direct proportion to the demands placed upon them, a basic principle of muscle physiology. The final principle was *progressive intensity*, an escalation of exercise magnitude and degree of difficulty over time, key to increasing PFM strength and endurance.

WHO KNEW? *Education = empowerment. Through education and focused, disciplined, sustained and progressive exercise, pelvic health can be restored. This is simply a case of tapping into your body's remarkable ability to adapt to the stresses placed upon it.*

The Kegel Device—The Perineometer

Kegel created this special apparatus that provided resistance and measured PFM strength in order to help restore pelvic function and tone in women who had recently delivered babies.

The *perineometer* is a pneumatic chamber about 3 inches in length and less than 1 inch in width that fits inside the vagina. It is attached by tubing to a pressure-measuring tool (similar to a blood pressure gadget) capable of measuring a pressure ranging from 0-100 millimeters (mm). The patient inserted the device into her vagina and then performed PFM contractions. The device provided resistance to clench down upon, similar to contracting one's biceps against the resistance of the weight of a dumbbell as opposed to doing arm flexes with no weights. The perineometer allowed the user to observe the magnitude of each contraction of the PFM.

WHO KNEW? *In terms of feedback, the Kegel pressure-measuring device is not unlike the "ring the bell" strongman game at an amusement park where one swings a mallet as hard as they can in an effort to ring a bell mounted at the top.*

This feedback element was of vital importance to the PFMT process, serving as a visual aid and confirming to the patient that the proper muscles were being contracted. It also served the purpose of showing day-to-day improvement, helping to encourage the participant to complete the program. Kegel recommended recording the maximal contraction at each exercise session, the written documentation providing further encouragement.

WHO KNEW? *Tracking one's performance is fundamental to the success of PFMT. By being able to observe forward progress over time, the process is enabled.*

Kegel observed that when the vaginal muscles were well developed and had a contractile strength of 20 mm or more, sexual complaints were infrequent. However, when the vaginal muscles were thin, poorly toned, inelastic and had a weak contractile strength of 0-3 mm, sexual dissatisfaction was commonplace. Kegel observed that younger patients progressed more rapidly through PFMT than older ones.

WHO KNEW? *Patients vary greatly in their ability to contract their vaginal muscles. Some women are incapable of clenching down on an examining finger in the vagina, whereas others can squeeze so hard that the finger hurts!*

Kegel recognized that reconditioning the PFM proceeded in a sequence of stages. The initial phase was *awareness and coordination.* The next phase was *transitional,* the adaptive phase when the body learns how to properly execute the exercises; this was followed by *regeneration,* when the PFM respond to the exercises and increase their mass, strength, power and coordination. The final stage was *restoration,* in which there is a leveling out of the maximal PFM contractions.

WHO KNEW? *Kegel observed that following restoration of pelvic floor muscle function in women with incontinence or pelvic laxity, many patients had increased sexual feelings—including more readily achieved and better quality orgasms.*

Kegel's PFMT regimen was rigorous, requiring a significant investment of time: 20 minutes three times daily for a total of 20-40 hours of progressive resistance exercise over a 20-60 day period. He emphasized the importance of not only doing PFMT after pregnancy, but also prophylactically during pregnancy.

Note: The same successful outcomes that Kegel obtained with his PFMT regimen can be achieved with PFMT programs that are less time consumptive and physically demanding. Forthcoming chapters provide specially designed exercises—based upon Dr. Kegel's principles—that strengthen the PFM and address the specific pelvic floor dysfunctions in an efficient and effective manner.

4 TWELVE MYTHS ABOUT KEGEL EXERCISES

Myth 1 **The best way to do Kegels is to stop the flow of urine.**

Truth: If you can stop your stream, it is proof that you are contracting the proper muscles. However, this is just a means of *feedback* to reinforce that you are employing the right muscles. The bathroom should not be your PFM gymnasium!

Myth 2 **Do Kegel exercises as often as possible.**

Truth: PFMT strengthens and tones the PFM and like other muscle-conditioning routines, should not be performed every day. PFMT should be done in accordance with a structured plan of progressively more difficult and challenging exercises that require rest periods in order for optimal muscle growth and response.

Myth 3 **Do Kegels anywhere (stopped at a red light, waiting in line at the supermarket, while watching television, etc.).**

Truth: Exercises of the PFM—like any other form of exercise—demand attention, mindfulness and isolation of the muscle group. Until you are able to master the exercise regimen, it is best that the exercises be performed in an appropriate venue, free of distraction, which allows single-minded focus and concentration. This is not to say that once you achieve mastery of the exercises and a fit pelvic floor that you should not integrate the exercises into activities of daily living. That, in fact, is one of the goals.

Myth 4   The best way to do a Kegel contraction is to squeeze your PFM as hard as you can.

Truth: A good quality Kegel contraction takes the PFM through the full range of motion from maximal relaxation to maximal contraction. The relaxation element is as critical as the contraction element. As vital as "tone and tighten" are, "stretch and lengthen" are of equal importance. The goal is for PFM that are strong, toned, supple and *flexible*.

Myth 5   Keeping the PFM tightly contracted all the time is desirable.

Truth: This is not a good idea. The PFM have a natural resting tone to them and when you are not actively engaging and exercising them, they should be left to their own natural state. "Tight" is not the same as "strong." There exists a condition—PFM tension myalgia—in which there is spasticity, extreme tightness and pain due to excessive tension of these muscles.

Myth 6   Focusing on your core muscles is sufficient to ensure PFM fitness.

Truth: No. The PFM are the floor of the "core" group of muscles and get a workout whenever the core muscles are exercised. However, for maximum benefit, specific focus needs to be made on the PFM. In Pilates and yoga, there is an emphasis on the core group of muscles and a collateral benefit to the PFM, but this is not enough to achieve the full potential fitness of a regimen that focuses exclusively and intensively on the PFM.

Myth 7   Kegel exercises do not help.

Truth: Oh yes they do . . . PFMT has been medically proven to help a variety of pelvic maladies including urinary and bowel incontinence, pelvic relaxation and sexual dysfunction. Additionally, PFMT will improve core strength and stability, posture and spinal alignment.

Myth 8   Kegels are only helpful after a problem arises.

Truth: No, no, no. As in any exercise regimen, the best option is to be proactive and not reactive. It is sensible to optimize muscle mass, strength and endurance to prevent problems from surfacing before they have an opportunity to do so. PFMT undertaken before getting pregnant will aid in preventing pelvic issues that may arise as a consequence of pregnancy, labor and delivery. If you strengthen the PFM when you are young, you can help avoid pelvic, urinary and bowel conditions that may arise as you age. Strengthen and tone now and your body will thank you later.

Myth 9   You can stop doing Kegels once your muscles strengthen.

Truth: Not true . . . the "use it or lose it" principle applies here as it does in any muscle-training regimen. Just as muscles adapt positively to the stresses and resistances placed upon them, so they adapt negatively to a lack of stresses and resistances. "Disuse atrophy" is a possibility with all muscles, including the PFM. "Maintenance" PFMT should be used after completing a course of PFMT.

Myth 10   It is easy to learn how to isolate and exercise the PFM.

Truth: Not the case at all. A high percentage of women who think they are doing PFM exercises properly are actually contracting other muscles or are bearing down and straining instead of drawing up and in. However, with a little instruction and effort you can become the master of your pelvic domain.

Myth 11   Kegels are bad for your sex life.

Truth: Just the opposite! PFMT improves sexual function as the PFM play a critical role in genital blood flow and lubrication, vaginal tone, clitoral erection and orgasm. Kegels will enhance your sex life and his as well. Strong PFM will enable you to "hug" his penis as energetically as you can hug his body with your arms!

Myth 12   Kegels are just for women.

Truth: Au contraire . . . men have essentially the same PFM as do women and can reap similar benefits from PFMT with respect to sexual, urinary and bowel health. For more information on this topic, refer to *Male Pelvic Fitness: Optimizing Sexual and Urinary Health (www.MalePelvicFitness.com)*.

Note: Chapters 5-11 address those specific PFM dysfunctions that PFMT can benefit. Chapters 12-14 spell out the details of the various PFMT programs.

5

PELVIC ORGAN PROLAPSE (POP)

Tap into the powers of your PFM to improve pelvic organ prolapse.

The thought was delivered just after my newborn's placenta: A sneaking suspicion that things were not quite the same down there, and they might never be again. I was reminded of the kGoal, a device that claimed it could tone my ladyparts back into pre-baby shape. Once my daughter had finished using my vagina as a giant elastic waterslide, I knew I had to try it.

—Alissa Walker, "I Toned My Weak Vagina With This Little Blue Blob," Gizmodo.com, April 2, 2015

Introduction

The female bony pelvis provides the infrastructure to support the pelvic organs and to allow childbirth. Adequate "closure" is needed for pelvic organ support, yet sufficient "opening" is necessary to permit vaginal delivery. The female pelvis evolved as a compromise between these two important, but opposing functions.

WHO KNEW? *When humans evolved from four legs to two legs, it created the need for adaptation of pelvic floor support to accommodate the forces on the pelvic floor that are very much different in the upright position.*

WHO KNEW? *The supportive function of the PFM is an acquired function that develops when infants become capable of standing. At that time, the PFM become the true floor of the pelvic cavity. With assumption of erect posture, the PFM adapt the capacity for pelvic organ support.*

The PFM divide the abdominal and pelvic cavities above from the perineum below, forming an important structural support system that keeps the pelvic organs in place. Many physical activities result in significant increases in abdominal pressure, the force of which is largely exerted downwards towards the pelvic floor, especially when upright. This pelvic floor "loading" puts the PFM at particular risk for damage with the potential for pelvic organ prolapse (POP), a.k.a. pelvic relaxation or pelvic organ hernia.

WHO KNEW? *Gravity contributes in a major way to POP, a situation in which the pelvic organs go wayward, literally "popping" out of place.*

POP is a common condition in which there is weakness of the PFM and other connective tissues that provide pelvic support, allowing the pelvic organs to move from their normal positions into the space of the vaginal canal and, at its most severe degree, outside the vaginal opening. Chances are that if you have delivered a child vaginally, you have some degree of relaxation of pelvic support, although you might not be aware of it. Two thirds of women who have delivered children have anatomical evidence of POP (although most are not symptomatic) and 10-20% will need to undergo a corrective surgical procedure.

POP is not life threatening, but can be a distressing and disruptive problem that negatively impacts quality of life. Despite how common an issue it is, many women are reluctant to seek help because they are too embarrassed to discuss it with anyone or have the misconception that there are no treatment options available or fear that surgery will be the only solution.

POP may involve any of the pelvic organs including those of the urinary, intestinal and gynecological tracts. The bladder is the organ that is most commonly involved in POP. POP can vary from minimal descent—causing few, if any, symptoms—to major descent—in which one or more of the pelvic organs prolapse outside the vagina at all times, causing significant symptoms. The degree of descent varies with position and activity level, increasing with the upright position and/or exertion and decreasing with lying down and resting, as is the case for any hernia.

WHO KNEW? *POP often causes a bulge outside the vaginal opening, appearing like a man's scrotum. Little wonder why most women are disturbed by this condition!*

POP can give rise to a variety of symptoms, depending on which organ is involved and the extent of the prolapse. The most common complaints are the following: a vaginal bulge or lump, the perception that one's insides are falling outside, and vaginal "pressure." Because POP often causes vaginal looseness in addition to one or more organs falling into the space of the vaginal canal, sexual complaints are common, including painful intercourse, altered sexual feeling and difficulty achieving orgasm as well as less partner satisfaction.

Women with POP have lower genital sensitivity to vibration and temperature stimulation as compared to women without POP, suggesting that a sensory nerve deficit may be associated with POP.

When your bladder or rectum descends into the vaginal space, there can be an obstruction to the passage of urine or stool, respectively. This often requires placing one or more fingers in the vagina to manually push back the malpositioned organ. Doing so will straighten the "kink" in order to facilitate emptying your bladder or bowels. Your fingers do not necessarily need to remain inside the vagina while urinating or moving your bowels, although in those with greater extents of POP, it may be necessary. Pushing a prolapsed organ back into position with your finger(s) is called "splinting," an apt term since a splint is a device used for support and immobilization of a finger, limb or other body part.

WHO KNEW?   *If you have a prolapsed bladder, incontinence with sexual activity can occur. Upon vaginal penetration the penis displaces the bladder back into its normal anatomic position and relieves the obstruction, resulting in urinary leakage. This does not make for a happy couple.*

WHO KNEW?   *The laxity of the PFM that causes POP can on occasion provide the means for air to enter the vagina, resulting in what is referred to as "vaginal flatulence," which can be a noisy and embarrassing condition.*

Causes Of POP

POP results from a combination of factors including multiple pregnancies and vaginal deliveries (especially deliveries of large babies), menopause, hysterectomy, aging and weight gain. Additionally, conditions that give rise to chronic increases in abdominal pressure contribute to POP. These include asthma, bronchitis and emphysema (chronic wheezing and coughing), seasonal allergies (chronic sneezing), chronic constipation and repetitive heavy lifting, whether work-associated or due to weight training. Other causes are genetic predispositions to POP and connective tissue disorders.

Childbirth is one of the most traumatic events that the female body experiences and vaginal delivery is the single most important factor in the development of POP. Passage of the large human head through the female pelvis causes intense mechanical pressure and tissue trauma (stretching, tearing, compression and crushing) to the PFM and PFM nerve supply. This results in separation or weakness of connective tissue attachments and alterations and damage to the integrity of the pelvis. POP that occurs because of a difficult vaginal delivery may not manifest until decades later. It is unusual for women who have not had children or who have delivered by elective caesarian section to develop significant POP.

Pelvic injuries sustained during childbirth can take many months or longer to heal. MRI imaging studies demonstrate that about 15% of women sustain pelvic trauma that fails to heal, including the following injuries: fluid within the marrow of the pelvic bones; pelvic bone stress fractures; excessive fluid within muscles indicative of severe muscle strains; and PFM tears and detachments from the pelvic bones.

Chronic constipation is a major risk factor in perpetuating POP since it is equivalent to being in "labor" on an everyday basis. Menopause is also a significant factor for furthering POP because of declining levels of the female hormone estrogen, which negatively affects pelvic tissue integrity, strength and elasticity. Neuromuscular diseases that negatively impact muscle strength can contribute to POP. Hysterectomy is a risk factor for POP with more than 10% of women after hysterectomy requiring a second operation for POP. After removal of the uterus, weakness of the deep support tissues of the vagina may develop, allowing small intestine to occupy the space once filled by the uterus. This type of small intestinal POP is known as "enterocele," and is often accompanied by POP of the vagina itself, a condition in which the vagina turns inside out.

Organs Affected by POP

The defect in POP is not with the pelvic organ per se, but with the tissue support of that organ. POP is not the problem, but the result of the problem. The prolapsed organ is merely an "innocent passenger" in the POP process.

POP can involve one or more of the pelvic organs including the following: urethra (*urethral hypermobility*); bladder (*cystocele*); rectum (*rectocele*); uterus (*uterine prolapse*); intestines (*enterocele*); the vagina itself (*vaginal vault prolapse*); and the perineum (*perineal laxity*).

The simplest system for grading POP severity uses a scale of 1-4: 1 (slight POP); grade 2 (POP to vaginal opening with straining); grade 3 (POP beyond vaginal opening with straining); grade 4 (POP beyond vaginal opening without straining).

WHO KNEW? *The vagina can be simplistically thought of as a box that is closed on all sides but one. The open end is the vaginal opening and the opposite end is the deepest part of the vagina (apex). This defines three compartments: the roof (anterior compartment), the closed deep end (apical compartment) and the floor (posterior compartment). The urethra and bladder sit above the roof and potentially can prolapse into the anterior compartment. The rectum sits below the floor and potentially can prolapse into the posterior compartment. The cervix and uterus sit in the apex and potentially can prolapse into the apical compartment. Vault prolapse occurs when the entire box becomes unmoored and flips inside out.*

Urethra

When the support structures of the urethra are weak, a sudden increase in abdominal pressure (from a cough, sneeze, jump or other physical exertion) will push the urethra down and out of its normal position, a condition known as *urethral hypermobility*. With no effective "backboard" of support tissue under the urethra, stress urinary incontinence will often occur. Chapter 8 is dedicated to this topic.

WHO KNEW? *The healthy well-supported urethra has a "backboard" or "hammock" of support tissue that lies beneath it. With a sudden increase in abdominal pressure, the urethra is pushed downwards, but because of the backboard's presence, the urethra gets pinched closed between the abdominal pressure above and the hammock below, allowing for normal continence.*

Bladder

Descent of the bladder through a weakness in its supporting tissues gives rise to a cystocele, a.k.a. "dropped bladder," "prolapsed bladder," or "bladder hernia." A *central* cystocele occurs when the bladder falls into the roof of the vagina as a result of a weakness of the PFM and connective tissues between the top wall of the vagina and the bladder. A *lateral* cystocele occurs when the attachment of the bladder to the pelvic sidewalls weakens.

Cystoceles typically cause one or more of the following symptoms:

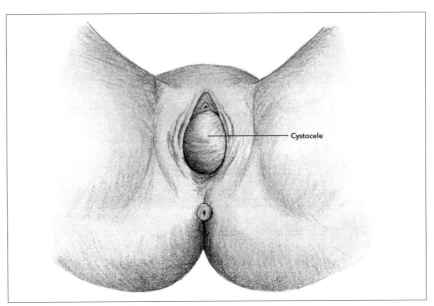

Figure 4. Pelvic Organ Prolapse

a bulge or lump protruding into or even outside the vagina; the need for pushing the cystocele back in in order to urinate; obstructive urinary symptoms (a slow, weak stream that stops and starts and incomplete bladder emptying) due to the prolapsed bladder causing urethral kinking; irritative urinary symptoms (frequent and urgent urinating); and vaginal pain and/or painful intercourse.

Even though the bladder and urethra can be thought of as one unit, in reality the degree of support of each can differ. The urinary symptoms of a cystocele are variable and depend upon the relative support of the bladder and urethra. When the urethral support is less adequate than the bladder support, stress urinary incontinence often occurs. When bladder support is less adequate than urethral support, a kinking phenomenon can occur, often resulting in obstructive urinary symptoms. The bottom line is that the specifics of the anatomical changes determine the functional problems that result.

Rectum

Descent of the rectum through a weakness in its supporting tissues gives rise to a rectocele, a.k.a. "dropped rectum," "prolapsed rectum," or "rectal hernia." The rectum protrudes into the floor of the vagina because of a weakness in the PFM and connective tissues between the floor of the vagina and the rectum.

Rectoceles typically cause one or more of the following symptoms: a bulge or lump protruding into the vagina, especially noticeable during bowel movements; a kink of the normally straight rectum causing difficulty with bowel movements and the need for vaginal splinting to empty the bowels; incomplete emptying of the rectum; fecal incontinence; and vaginal pain and/or painful intercourse.

WHO KNEW? *The word "rectum" is from the Latin word meaning "straight," because under normal circumstances the rectum is a straight chute, facilitating bowel movements. A rectocele allows a kink of the rectum to occur, destroying this anatomical arrangement and making bowel movements difficult without splinting the rectum using one or more fingers placed in the vagina.*

Perineum

Often accompanying a rectocele is perineal muscle laxity, a condition in which the superficial PFM (those located in the region between the vagina and anus) become flabby. Weakness in these PFM cause the following anatomical changes: a widened and loose vaginal opening, decreased distance between the vagina and anus, and a change in the vaginal axis such that the vagina assumes a more upwards orientation as opposed to its normal downwards angulation towards the sacral bones.

Vaginal laxity is not caused by an intrinsic problem with the vagina, but by the extrinsic weakened PFM that no longer provide optimal vaginal support.

Women with this issue who are sexually active may complain of a loose or gaping vagina, making intercourse less satisfying for themselves and their partners. This may lead to difficulty achieving orgasm, difficulty retaining tampons, difficulty retaining the penis with vaginal intercourse, the vagina filling with water while bathing and vaginal flatulence. The perception of having a loose vagina can often lead to low self-esteem.

WHO KNEW? *Women with POP who have an enlarged vaginal outlet from obstetrical trauma and other factors often have difficulty in properly "accommodating" the penis, resulting in the vagina "surrounding" the penis rather than firmly "squeezing" it, with the end result being diminished sensation for both partners.*

WHO KNEW? *Under normal circumstances, sexual intercourse results in indirect clitoral stimulation. The clitoral shaft moves rhythmically with penile thrusting by virtue of penile traction on the inner vaginal lips, which join together to form the hood of the clitoris. However, if the vaginal opening is too wide to permit the penis to put enough traction on* *the inner vaginal lips, there will be limited clitoral stimulation and less satisfaction in the bedroom.*

WHO KNEW? *Leonardo Da Vinci made an interesting observation on perspectives: "Woman's desire is the opposite of that of man. She wishes the size of the man's member to be as large as possible, while the man desires the opposite for the woman's genital parts."*

Small Intestine

The *peritoneum* is a thin sac that contains the abdominal organs, including the small intestine. Descent of the peritoneal contents through a weakness in the supporting tissues at the innermost part of the vagina (the apex of the vagina) gives rise to an *enterocele*, a.k.a. "dropped small intestine," "small intestine prolapse," or "small intestine hernia."

Enteroceles typically cause one or more of the following symptoms: a bulge or lump protruding through the vagina, intestinal cramping due to small intestine trapped within the enterocele, and vaginal pressure/pain and/or painful intercourse.

WHO KNEW? *On pelvic exam an enterocele has a characteristic tongue-like appearance.*

Uterus

Descent of the uterus and cervix because of weakness of their supporting structures results in uterine prolapse, a.k.a. "dropped uterus," "prolapsed uterus," or "uterine hernia." Normally, the cervix is situated deeply in the vagina. As uterine prolapse progresses, the extent of descent into the vaginal canal will increase.

Uterine POP typically causes one or more of the following symptoms: a bulge or lump protruding from the vagina; difficulty urinating; the need to manually push back the uterus in order to urinate; urinary urgency and frequency; urinary incontinence; kidney obstruction because of the descent of the bladder and ureters (tubes that drain urine from the kidneys to the bladder) that are dragged down with the uterus, creating a kink of the ureters; vaginal pain with sitting and walking; painful intercourse; and spotting and/or bloody vaginal discharge from the malpositioned uterus, which becomes subject to trauma and abrasions from being out of position.

WHO KNEW? *The most extreme form of uterine POP is uterine "procidentia," a situation in which the uterus is exteriorized at all times and, because of external exposure, has a tendency for ulceration and bleeding.*

Vaginal Vault

The most advanced stage of POP occurs when the support structures of the vagina are weakened to such an extent that the vaginal canal itself turns inside out. Vault prolapse, a.k.a. "dropped vaginal vault," "prolapsed vaginal vault," or "vaginal vault hernia," is rarely an isolated event, but often occurs in association with other forms of POP and most often is a consequence of hysterectomy.

WHO KNEW?   *If the vagina is likened to an internal "sock," vaginal vault prolapse is a condition in which the sock is turned inside out. When I explain vaginal vault prolapse to patients, I demonstrate it by turning a front pocket of my pants inside out.*

Diagnosis of POP

After obtaining a thorough verbal history, the next step is a pelvic examination with the patient's legs in stirrups. The problem with examining a female in this position is that this is NOT the position in which POP typically manifests itself, POP being a problem of standing and exertion. For this reason, the exam must be performed with the patient straining forcefully enough to demonstrate the POP at its fullest extent.

A thorough pelvic examination involves visual observation, a single blade speculum exam, passage of a small catheter into the bladder and a digital exam. Each region of potential prolapse through the vagina—roof, apex, floor—must be examined independently.

Inspection will determine tissue integrity and the presence of a vaginal bulge with straining. After menopause, typical changes include thinning of the vaginal skin, redness, irritation, etc. The ridges and folds within the vagina that are typical in younger women tend to disappear after menopause.

WHO KNEW?   *The normal vulva is shut like a closed clam. POP often causes the vaginal lips to gape like an open clam.*

Since the vagina has top and bottom walls and since the bulge-like appearance of POP of the bladder or rectum look virtually identical—like a red rubber ball—it is important to use a single blade speculum to sort out which organ is prolapsing and to determine its extent. A single blade speculum is used to pull down the bottom wall of the vagina to observe the top wall for the presence of urethral hypermobility and cystocele, and likewise, to pull up the top wall to inspect for the presence of rectocele and perineal laxity. To examine for uterine prolapse and enterocele, both top and bottom walls must be pulled up and down, respectively, using two single blade specula. Once the speculum is placed, the patient is asked to strain vigorously and comparisons are made between the extent of POP resting and straining.

After the patient has emptied her bladder, a small catheter (a narrow hollow straw-like tube) is passed into the bladder to determine how much urine remains in the bladder, to submit a urine culture in the event that urinalysis suggests a urinary infection and to determine urethral angulation. With the catheter in place, the angle that the urethra makes with the horizontal is measured. The catheter is typically parallel with the horizontal at rest. The patient is asked to strain and the angulation is again measured, recording the change in urethral angulation that occurs between resting and straining. Urethral angulation with straining (hypermobility) is a sign of loss of urethral support, which often causes SUI.

Finally, a digital examination is performed to assess vaginal tone and PFM strength. A bimanual exam (combined internal and external exam in which the pelvic organs are felt between vaginal and external examining fingers) is done to check for the presence of pelvic masses.

WHO KNEW? *On pelvic exam it is usually very obvious whether or not a woman has had vaginal deliveries. The pelvic support and tone of the vagina in a woman who has not delivered vaginally can usually be described as "high and tight," as opposed to "low and loose" in a woman who has had multiple vaginal deliveries.*

Depending upon circumstances, tests to further evaluate POP may be used, including an endoscopic inspection of the lining of the bladder and urethra (cystoscopy), sophisticated functional tests of bladder storage and emptying (urodynamics) and, on occasion, imaging tests (bladder fluoroscopy or pelvic MRI).

The ideal position to examine a woman with POP is standing, but this obviously is difficult and awkward. For this reason, if a woman is diagnosed with a cystocele, an informative test is imaging the contrast-filled bladder at rest and with straining and coughing in the upright position using fluoroscopy (x-ray video watched on a screen in real time, not requiring the taking and developing of x-ray photographs). This is useful to determine the specific type and extent of cystocele. On fluoroscopy, the normal, well-supported bladder appears oval in shape. The "central defect" cystocele appears like the handle of a ping pong racquet as opposed to the "lateral defect" cystocele, which has a triangular appearance. Many women are found to have a "combined" cystocele, with elements of both central and lateral defects.

Management of POP

There are three means of managing POP: conservative treatments, pessaries and surgery (pelvic reconstruction).

Conservative treatment options for POP include PFMT, modification of activities that promote the POP (heavy lifting and high impact exercises), management of constipation and other circumstances that increase abdominal pressure, weight loss, smoking cessation and consideration for hormone replacement, since estrogen replacement can increase tissue integrity and suppleness.

Pessaries are mechanical devices that are available in a variety of sizes and shapes and are inserted into the vagina to act as "struts" to help provide pelvic support. The side effects of pessaries are vaginal infection and discharge, the inability to retain the pessary in proper position, and SUI, caused by the "unmasking" of the incontinence that occurs when the prolapsed bladder is splinted back into position by the pessary. Pessaries need to be removed periodically in order to clean them. Some are designed to permit sexual intercourse.

Studies comparing the use of pessaries with PFMT in managing women with advanced POP have shown that both can significantly improve symptoms; however, PFMT was more effective specifically for bladder POP.

PFMT for POP

Note: The specifics of the PFMT program tailored for POP are covered in Chapter 13.

PFMT is useful under the circumstances of mild-moderate POP, for those who cannot or do not want to have surgery and for those whose minimal symptoms do not warrant more aggressive options. The goal of PFMT is to increase the strength, tone and endurance of the PFM that play a key role in the support of the pelvic organs. Weak PFM can be strengthened; however, if POP is due to connective tissue damage, PFMT will not remedy the injury, but will strengthen the PFM that can help compensate for the connective tissue impairment. PFMT is most effective in women with lesser degrees of POP and chances are that if your POP is moderate-severe, PFMT will be less effective. However, if not cured, the POP can still be improved, and that might be sufficient for you.

Numerous scientific studies have demonstrated the benefits of PFMT for POP, including improved PFM strength, pelvic support and a reduction in the severity and symptoms of POP. Improvements in pelvic support via PFMT are most notable with bladder POP as opposed to rectal or uterine POP. PFMT is also capable of preventing POP from developing when applied to a healthy female population without POP.

In symptomatic advanced POP, surgery is often necessary, particularly when quality of life has been significantly impacted. There are a number of considerations that go into the decision-making process regarding the specifics of the surgical procedure (pelvic reconstruction) to improve/cure the problem. These factors include which organ or organs are prolapsed; the extent and severity of the POP; the desire to have children in the future; the desire to be sexually active; age; and, if the POP involves a cystocele, the specific type of cystocele (since there are different approaches depending on the type). Surgery to repair POP can be performed vaginally or abdominally (open, laparoscopic or robotic), and can be done with or without mesh (synthetic netting or other biological materials used to reinforce the repair). The goal of surgery is restoration of normal anatomy with preservation of vaginal length, width and axis and improvement in symptoms with optimization of bladder, bowel and sexual function.

More than 300,000 surgical procedures for repair of POP are performed annually in the United States. An estimated 10-20% of women will undergo an operation for POP over the course of their lifetime.

Kegel believed that surgical procedures for female incontinence and pelvic relaxation are facilitated by pre-operative and post-operative PFM exercises. Like cardiac rehabilitation after cardiac surgery and physical rehabilitation after orthopedic procedures, PFMT after pelvic reconstruction surgery can help minimize recurrences. Pre-operative PFMT—as advocated by Kegel—can sometimes improve pelvic support to an extent such that surgery will not be necessary. At the very least, proficiency of the PFM learned pre-operatively (before surgical incisions are made and pelvic anatomy is altered) will make the process of post-operative rehabilitation that much easier.

WHO KNEW? *Sherrie Palm is an advocate, champion and crusader for women's pelvic health who has made great strides with respect to POP awareness, guidance and support. She is founder and director of the Association for Pelvic Organ Prolapse Support and author of "Pelvic Organ Prolapse: The Silent Epidemic." Visit PelvicOrganProlapseSupport.org.*

6

SEX AND THE PFM

Tap into the powers of your PFM to improve your
sexual pleasure (as well as that of your partner).

*A healthy pelvic floor--one with well-toned muscles capable of going
through their full range of motion, with a healthy blood flow nour-
ishing healthy tissue, with nerve cells that respond well to stimula-
tion--has all ingredients necessary to ensure sensitivity to stimulation,
powerful arousal and a highly satisfying climax.*

—Amy Stein, *Heal Pelvic Pain*

Introduction

Sex is a fundamental human need, a powerful means of connecting and
bonding that is central to the intimacy of interpersonal relationships,
contributing to well being and overall quality of life. Healthy sexual
functioning is a vital part of general, physical, mental, social and emotional health.

Female sexuality is a complex and dynamic process involving the in-
terplay of anatomical, physiological, hormonal, psychological, emotional and cultural factors that impact desire, arousal, lubrication and
orgasm. Although desire is biologically driven based on one's internal
hormonal environment, many psychological and emotional factors play
into it as well. Arousal requires erotic and/or physical stimulation that
results in increased pelvic blood flow, which causes genital engorgement,
vaginal lubrication and vaginal anatomical changes that allow the vagina
to accommodate an erect penis. The ability to orgasm depends on the

occurrence of a sequence of physiological and emotional responses, culminating in involuntary rhythmic contractions of the PFM.

WHO KNEW? *The sexual research by Masters and Johnson demonstrated that the primary reaction to sexual stimulation is vaso-congestion (increased blood flow) and the secondary reaction is an increase in muscle tension. Orgasm is the release from the state of vaso-congestion and muscle tension.*

The PFM play a pivotal role with respect to sexual function, their contractions facilitating and enhancing sexual response. They contribute to arousal, sensation during intercourse and the ability to clench the vagina and firmly "grip" the penis. The strength and durability of PFM contractions are directly related to orgasmic potential since the PFM are the "motor" that drives sexual climax.

WHO KNEW? *Supple and pliable PFM with trampoline-like tone are capable of a "pulling up and in" action that will put some bounce into your sex life ... and that of your partner!*

Female sexual dysfunction is a common problem, affecting up to 55% of women and causing significant emotional distress. It can take many forms: decreased sexual desire; impaired emotional arousal or genital arousal with insufficient lubrication; delayed orgasm or inability to orgasm; and painful sexual intercourse. Sexuality goes way beyond simply having a functional vagina since the vagina does not act in isolation, its function contributed to and affected by biological, psychological, social and emotional factors.

The most common female sexual dysfunction is low sexual desire, a.k.a. Hypoactive Sexual Desire Disorder (HSDD) in medical lingo. It is defined as deficiency or absence of erotic thoughts, fantasies, and/or desire for or receptivity to sexual activity, which can cause marked personal distress and/or interpersonal issues.

WHO KNEW? *In August 2015, the FDA approved the first prescription drug to enhance women's sex drive. Addyi (Flibanserin) is thought to increase libido by altering the balance of brain neurotransmitters.*

PFM dysfunction can dramatically affect sexual function. From one extreme when the PFM are weak and/or poorly toned to the other extreme when the PFM are too tense, sexual function becomes compromised. PFM weakness often results in vaginal laxity, undermining sensation for both the female and her partner. On the other hand, when the PFM are too taut, sexual intercourse can be painful, if not impossible.

WHO KNEW? *Childbirth is one of the key culprits in causing weakened and stretched PFM, leading to loss of vaginal tone, diminished sensation with sexual stimulation and impaired ability to tighten the vagina.*

Pelvic organ prolapse can reduce sexual gratification on a mechanical basis from vaginal laxity and uncomfortable or painful intercourse. However, the psychological impact goes way beyond the physical, including a negative image of one's vagina, insecurity about partner satisfaction, embarrassment, feeling unattractive, depression, etc., all of which can negatively affect sexual fulfillment. The body image issues that result from vaginal laxity and POP are profound and may be the most important factors that diminish one's sex life. As the pelvic floor loses strength and tone, there is often an accompanying loss of sexual confidence.

Urinary incontinence can also contribute to an unsatisfying sex life because of fears of leakage during intercourse, concerns about odor and not feeling clean, embarrassment about the need for pads, and a negative body image perception. This can adversely influence sex drive, arousal and ability to orgasm.

A healthy sexual response involves being "in the moment," free of concerns and worries. Women with incontinence and/or pelvic organ prolapse are often mentally distracted during intercourse, preoccupied with their lack of control over their problem as well as their perception of their vagina being "not normal" and what consequences this might have on their partner's sexual experience.

A Few Words on Genital Embryology

WHO KNEW? *Female and male external genitals are remarkably similar. In fact, in the first few weeks of existence as an embryo, the external genitals are identical.*

The female external genitals are the "default" model, which will remain female in the absence of the male hormone *testosterone*. In this circumstance, the *genital tubercle* (a midline swelling) becomes the clitoris; the *urogenital folds* (two vertically-oriented folds of tissue below the genital tubercle) become the labia minora (inner lips); and the *labio-scrotal swellings* (two vertically-oriented bulges outside the urogenital folds) fuse to become the labia majora (outer lips). In the presence of testosterone, the *genital tubercle* morphs into the penis; the *urogenital folds* fuse and become the urethra and part of the shaft of the penis; and the *labio-scrotal swellings* fuse to become the scrotal sac.

WHO KNEW?   *Your clitoris and his penis are essentially the same structure, as are your outer labia and his scrotum.*

Vulvas, Vestibules, Vaginas and More

WHO KNEW?   *When it comes to female genital anatomy, there are an abundance of words starting with the letter "V". What could be a better choice since the vulva is V-shaped?*

WHO KNEW?   *The hidden nether parts are a real mystery zone to a surprising number of women, who have very poor knowledge of the inner workings of their own sexual anatomy. Many falsely believe that the "pee hole" and "vagina hole" are one and the same. What is between your thighs is more complicated than you think . . . . There are three openings as well as lips and swellings, glands, erectile tissue and muscles. Learn your lady parts, as knowledge is power!*

The Vulva

The vulva is the outside part of your genitals. It consists of the *mons pubis, labia majora, labia minora, vestibule, vaginal opening, urethral opening* and *clitoris*.

Figure 5. Vulva

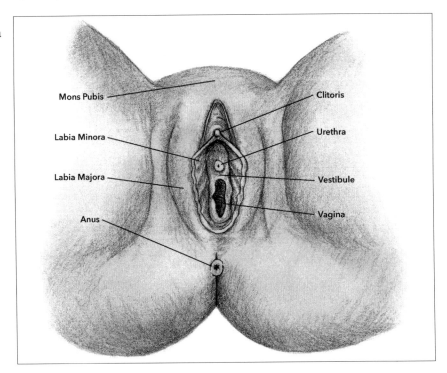

The mons pubis is the triangular mound that covers the pubic bone, consisting of hair-bearing skin and underlying fatty tissue. It extends down on each side to form the labia majora, folds of hair-bearing skin and underlying fatty tissue that surround the entrance to the vagina. Within the labia majora are two soft, hairless skin folds known as the labia minora, which safeguard the entrance to the vagina. The upper part of each labia minora unites to form the *clitoral hood* (*prepuce* or *foreskin*) at the upper part of the clitoris and the *frenulum* (a small band of tissue that secures the clitoral head to the hood) at the underside of the clitoris.

Who Knew?   *Labioplasty—a surgical procedure to trim the inner lips—has become one of the most common gynecological plastic surgery operations. Overly large labia minora can cause discomfort with tight clothes, exercise and sexual intercourse and can sometimes get caught in a zipper and may be aesthetically unpleasing to women who possess them. The goals of labial aesthetic surgery are labia minora that are symmetrical, straight and narrow and do not protrude beyond the labia majora.*

The Vestibule

A vestibule is an "entryway" and in the context of female anatomy is the plate of tissue located between the inner lips that surrounds and contains the entrances to the vagina and the urethra. Urine exits from the urethral opening on the vestibule and not from the vaginal opening. There is a small amount of vestibule tissue that separates the urethral opening from the vaginal opening.

The Vagina

WHO KNEW?   *Put your hand on your crotch. That is your VULVA, not your VAGINA. Place a finger internally within the vaginal opening . . . that's the vagina! Most women (and men) think of the vagina as the external and internal female genitals when in fact it is just internal.*

WHO KNEW?   *The word "vagina" derives from the Latin word for "sheath," a cover for the blade of a knife or sword.*

For many men—and women for that matter—the vagina is a dark and mysterious place. Nonetheless, the vagina is truly an amazingly versatile and multifunctional organ. It is a sexual organ that allows entry of the penis, an inflow pathway and receptacle for semen, an outflow pathway for menstruation and a birth canal for the fetus. It is by no means simply a passive channel for the passage of the penis, semen, menses and the fetus, but an active and responsive passageway that has the capacity for both spontaneous and voluntary muscular contraction. The elasticity of the vagina is impressive, with the ability to stretch to accommodate a baby's head and then return to a relatively normal caliber.

Anatomically, the vagina is an internal tube surrounded by a layer of muscle and connective tissue, extending from the vulva to the uterus. The vaginal muscle is comprised of inner smooth muscle that is circular in orientation and outer smooth muscle that is oriented longitudinally. Contraction of the inner muscle tightens the vagina. Contraction of the outer muscle shortens and widens the vagina. The vagina is secured within a "bed" of powerful PFM, both superficial and deep.

WHO KNEW?   *There is great variety in the bulk, strength, power and voluntary control of the PFM that support the vagina. Some women are capable of powerfully "snapping" their vaginas, while others cannot even generate a weak flicker.*

The vagina is banana-shaped. When you are lying down, face up, the more external part of the vagina is straight, and the inner, deeper part angles down towards the sacral bones. The vagina has pleats and corrugations called *rugae* that maximize the elasticity and stretchiness of the vagina. They are accordion-like ruffles and ridges that supply texture, which increases friction for the penis during sexual intercourse. In a young woman they are prominent, but with aging tend to disappear.

WHO KNEW?   *Rugae are similar to tire tread. In young women they appear like deep grooves on a new tire, whereas in older women they appear like thinning tire tread, completely bald at their most extreme.*

Under normal circumstances, the vagina is not "primed" for sex and is little more prepared for intercourse than is a flaccid penis. The unstimulated vagina is a potential space in which the vaginal roof and floor touch. With sexual stimulation, the vaginal walls undergo a "sweating-like" reaction as a result of pelvic blood congestion, creating a slippery and glistening film. Most of the lubrication is based upon seepage from this increased blood flow, but some comes from *Bartholin's* and *Skene's* glands. Simultaneously, the vagina expands with lengthening and widening of its inner two-thirds and flattening of the rugae. The cervix and uterus pull back and up.

Bartholin's glands are paired, pea-size glands that drain just below and to each side of the vagina. During sexual arousal they secrete small drops of fluid, resulting in moistening of the opening of the vagina. Skene's glands are paired glands that drain just above and to each side of the urethral opening. They are the female equivalent of the male prostate gland and secrete fluid with arousal.

WHO KNEW? *"Squirting." At the time of climax, some women are capable of "ejaculating" fluid. The nature of this fluid has been controversial, thought by some to be hyper-lubrication and others to be Bartholin's and/or Skene's gland secretions. There are certain women who "ejaculate" very large volumes of fluid at climax and studies have shown this to be urine released because of an involuntary bladder contraction that can accompany orgasm.*

WHO KNEW? *The G-Spot—Named after German gynecologist Ernst Grafenberg, this was first described in 1950 and was believed to be an erogenous zone located on the top wall of the vagina, anatomically situated between the vagina and the urethra. Stimulation of this spot was thought to promote arousal and vaginal orgasm. There is little scientific support for the existence of the G-spot as a discrete anatomical entity; however, many women feel that they possess an area on the roof of the vagina that is a particularly sensitive pleasure zone. Although its existence remains controversial, the G-spot is certainly a powerful social phenomenon.*

The Clitoris

WHO KNEW? *The word clitoris derives from the Greek "kleitoris," meaning "little hill."*

The clitoris is uniquely an erectile organ that has as its express purpose sexual function, as opposed to the penis, which is a "multi-tasking" sexual, urinary and reproductive organ. The clitoris is the center of female sensual focus and is the most sensitive erogenous zone of the body, playing a vital role in sensation and orgasm.

WHO KNEW? *If an orgasm is thought of as an "earthquake," the clitoris is the "epicenter." The head of the clitoris, typically only the size of a pea, is a dense bundle of sensory nerve fibers, thought to have greater nerve density than any other body part.*

Like the penis, the clitoris is composed of an external visible part and an internal, deeper, "invisible" part. The inner part is known as the *crura* (legs), which are shaped like a wishbone with each side attached to the pubic arch as it descends and diverges. The visible part is located above the opening of the urethra, near the junction point of the inner lips. Similar to the penis, the clitoris has a *glans* (head), a *shaft* (body) and is covered by a hood of tissue that is the female equivalent of the *prepuce* (foreskin).

The shaft and crura contain erectile tissue, consisting of spongy sinuses that become engorged with blood at the time of sexual stimulation, resulting in clitoral engorgement and erection. The *clitoral bulbs* are additional erectile tissues that are sac-shaped and are situated between the crura. With sexual stimulation, they become full, plumping and tightening the vaginal opening. One can think of the crura and bulbs as the roots of a tree, hidden from view and extending deeply below the surface, yet fundamental to the support and function of the clitoral shaft and clitoral glans above, which can be thought of as the trunk of a tree.

When the clitoris is stimulated, the shaft expands with accompanying swelling of the glans. With increasing stimulation, clitoral retraction occurs, in which the clitoral shaft and glans withdraw from their overhanging position, pulling inwards against the pubic bone.

Possessing a clitoris may be the closest a woman will ever get to know what it is like to have a penis, as the clitoris is the female version of the penis. However, the clitoris is a much more subtle and mysterious organ, a curiosity to many women and men alike. It is similar to the penis in that it becomes engorged when stimulated and because of its concentration of nerve fibers, is the site where most orgasms are triggered. The glans is extremely sensitive and many women avoid direct clitoral glans stimulation, focusing instead on the clitoral shaft and mons pubis. Clitorises, like penises, come in all different sizes and shapes. A very large clitoris does not appear much different from a very small penis. The average length of the clitoral shaft including the glans is 0.8 inches with a range of 0.2-1.4 inches. The average width of the clitoral glans is 0.2 inches with a range of 0.1-0.4 inches.

WHO KNEW? *Size Matters. Location Matters. Studies comparing clitoral anatomy in orgasmic versus anorgasmic women using magnetic resonance imaging have demonstrated that a smaller clitoral glans and greater distance of the clitoral body from the vaginal opening is more common in the anorgasmic population. This suggests that a larger clitoris that is closer to the vagina is more likely to be stimulated during penetrative sexual intercourse.*

WHO KNEW? *Most sexual positions fail to directly stimulate the clitoris. It would behoove many men to gain some clitoral literacy ("cliteracy")!*

During sexual stimulation, the clitoris engorges and becomes erect. Two of the superficial PFM—the *bulbocavernosus* (BC) and *ischiocavernosus* (IC)—contract and compress the deep internal portions of the clitoris, maintaining blood pressures within the clitoral erection chambers that are significantly higher than systemic blood pressures.

The bulbocavernosus reflex (BCR) is a contraction of the BC and IC muscles (and other superficial PFM including the anal sphincter) that occurs when the clitoris is stimulated. The BCR is important for maintaining clitoral rigidity, since with each contraction of the BC and IC muscles there is a surge of blood flow to the clitoris, perpetuating clitoral engorgement and erection.

A Few Words on Orgasms

With sexual excitement and stimulation there is increased pelvic blood flow that causes vaginal lubrication as well as congestion and engorgement of the vulva, vagina and clitoris. The "orgasmic platform" is the Masters and Johnson's term for the outer third of the vagina with engorged inner lips, which they considered to be the "base" of pelvic blood congestion. With increasing stimulation and arousal, physical tension within the genitals gradually builds and once sufficient intensity and duration of sexual stimulation surpass a threshold, involuntary rhythmic muscular contractions occur of the PFM, the vagina, uterus and anus, followed by the release of accumulated erotic tension and a euphoric state. Thereafter, the genital engorgement and congestion subside, muscle relaxation occurs and a peaceful state of physical and emotional bliss and afterglow become apparent.

Orgasm is not only a genital response, but a total body reaction causing numerous muscles to go into involuntary spasm, including the facial muscles, resulting in grimacing. The PFM contract rhythmically: a total of 10-15 contractions typically occur with the first 3-5 contractions occurring at 0.8-second intervals, after which the interval between contractions lengthens and the intensity of the contractions decreases. The orgasmic response also includes flushing of the skin and elevation of heart rate, respiratory rate and blood pressure.

WHO KNEW? *At the 2014 meeting of the Sexual Medical Society of North America in Miami, I attended a lecture by Dr. Irwin Goldstein. He defined an orgasm as "a variable transient peak sensation of intense pleasure creating an altered state of consciousness, usually with an initiation accompanied by involuntary, rhythmic contractions of the pelvic striated circumvaginal musculature, often with concomitant uterine and anal contractions and myotonia that resolves the sexually induced vasocongestion and myotonia, generally with an induction of well-being and contentment." Wow ... that is a mouthful! An orgasm is certainly difficult to articulate in words, but it's one of those things that ... well, you just know what it is.*

WHO KNEW?   *"Lots of Ways to Skin a Cat." Orgasms can sometimes be achieved by non-genital stimulation. Some women can climax simply by erotic thoughts, others by breast stimulation or foot massage.*

WHO KNEW?   *"Persistent genital arousal disorder" is a rare sexual dysfunction characterized by unwanted, unremitting and intrusive arousal, genital engorgement and multiple orgasms without sexual interest or stimulation. It causes great distress to those suffering with it and there are no known effective treatments. It typically does not resolve after orgasm.*

WHO KNEW?   *"Penis Captivus." This is a rare condition in which a male's erect penis becomes stuck within a female's vagina. It is theorized to be on the basis of intense contractions of the PFM, causing the vaginal walls to clamp down and entrap the penis. It usually is a brief event and after female orgasm and/or male ejaculation, withdrawal becomes possible. However, it sometimes requires medical attention with a couple showing up in the emergency room tightly connected, like Siamese twins.*

The Aging Vagina

The estrogen-stimulated healthy vagina of a young adult female has a very different appearance than that of a female after menopause. Age-related changes of the vulva and vagina lead to dry, thinned and brittle tissues with loss of vaginal length and width, lubrication potential and expansive ability. Considering that nature's ultimate purpose of sex is for reproduction, perhaps it is not surprising that when the body is no longer capable of producing offspring, changes occur that affect the anatomy and function of the sexual apparatus. However, one should not despair because there are solutions, including PFMT and hormonal replacement therapy.

WHO KNEW?   *"Atrophic vaginitis"/"Senile atrophy." These are some of the terms used for the aging vagina. There are many such hurtful and cruel labels for female issues, including "frigid" for women who have difficulty in climaxing. A much kinder term for "senile atrophy" is "genitourinary syndrome of menopause" and a less disparaging term for "frigid" is "anorgasmic."*

WHO KNEW?   *"Use it or lose it." Sexual intercourse can be painful after menopause because of anatomical changes that result in difficulty in accommodating a penis. This is particularly the case if one has not*

*been sexually active on a habitual basis. Regular sexual activity is
vital for maintaining the ability to have ongoing satisfactory sexual
intercourse. Vaginal penetration increases pelvic and vaginal blood
flow, optimizing lubrication and elasticity, while orgasms tone and
strengthen the PFM that support vaginal function.*

Menopause is a significant risk factor for the occurrence of pelvic floor
dysfunction with anatomical and functional changes occurring as a result of reduced levels of the female hormone estrogen. The vestibule,
vagina, urethra and base of the urinary bladder have abundant estrogen
receptors that are no longer stimulated after menopause, resulting in
diminished tissue elasticity and integrity. The labia become less robust,
the vaginal opening retracts and the vaginal walls become thinner and
lose rugae. The skin of the vulva becomes paler, thinner and more frag-
ile.

Often accompanying the physical changes of menopause are diminished sexual desire, arousal and ability to achieve orgasm. Pain, burning, itching and irritation of the vulva and vagina—particularly after
sexual intercourse—are commonplace. Urinary changes include burning with urination, frequency and urgency and recurrent urinary infections.

WHO KNEW? *Under normal circumstances, healthy bacteria reside in the vagina.
After menopause, this vaginal bacterial ecosystem changes, which
can predispose one to urinary tract infections.*

WHO KNEW? *Vaginal estrogen creams can help manage pelvic floor dysfunctions
in post-menopausal women, including painful intercourse, overactive
bladder, stress urinary incontinence, pelvic organ prolapse, symptoms
due to genitourinary syndrome of menopause and recurrent urinary
tract infections. Additionally, because estrogen creams restore
suppleness to the vaginal tissues, they can be very useful both before
and after surgery for stress urinary incontinence and pelvic organ
prolapse.*

The Muscles of Love

*I am more a prose writer than a poet, but here is a short poem that I
have composed about the muscles of love:*

> *Limber hip rotators,*
> *A powerful cardio-core,*
> *But forget not*
> *The oft-neglected pelvic floor.*

Sex is a physical activity involving many muscles that coordinate with seamless efficiency. Sex is all about movement, a synchronized kinetic chain integrating core muscles and external hip rotators in which both pelvic thrusting and outward rotation of the hips work effectively together to forge a well-choreographed, dance-like motion. It is a given that cardiac (aerobic) conditioning is a prerequisite for any endurance athletic endeavor, including SEXercise.

Three muscle groups are vital for optimal sexual function—*core muscles*, which maintain stability and provide a solid platform to enable pelvic thrusting; *external hip rotators*, which rotate the thighs outward and are the motor behind pelvic thrusting; and the floor of the core muscles—the *PFM*, which permit tightening and relaxing of the vagina, support clitoral erection and contract rhythmically at the time of orgasm. When these muscles are in tiptop shape, sexual function is optimized.

To review, the core muscles are the cylinder of torso muscles that surround the innermost layer of the abdomen. They function as an internal corset and shock absorber. In Pilates they are aptly referred to as the "powerhouse," providing stability, alignment and balance, but also allowing the extremity muscles a springboard from which to push off and work effectively. It is impossible to use your limbs without engaging a solid core and, likewise, it is not possible to use your genitals effectively during sex without engaging the core muscles.

WHO KNEW?   *Coregasm. According to the book "The Coregasm Workout," 10% of women are capable of achieving an orgasm when doing core exercises. It most often occurs when challenging core exercises are pursued immediately after cardio exercises, resulting in core muscle fatigue. The orgasms are described as less intense, but more "tingly" than a sexually derived orgasm.*

Rotation of your hips is a vital element of sexual movement. The external rotators are a group of muscles responsible for lateral (side) rotation of your femur (thigh) bone in the hip joint. My medical school anatomy professor referred to this group of muscles as the "muscles of copulation." Included in this group are the powerful gluteal muscles of your buttocks.

WHO KNEW?   *Not only do your gluteal muscles give your bottom a nice shape, but they are also vital for pelvic thrusting power, a maneuver that makes sex more pleasurable for all parties.*

To reiterate, the PFM make up the floor of the core. The deep layer is the *levator ani* ("lift the anus"), consisting of the *pubococcygeus, pub-*

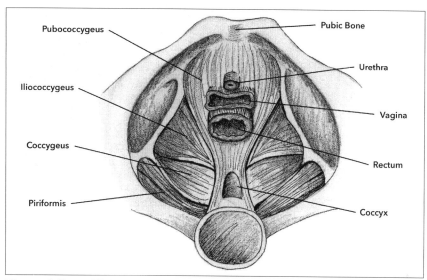

Figure 6. Deep PFM (Abdominal View)

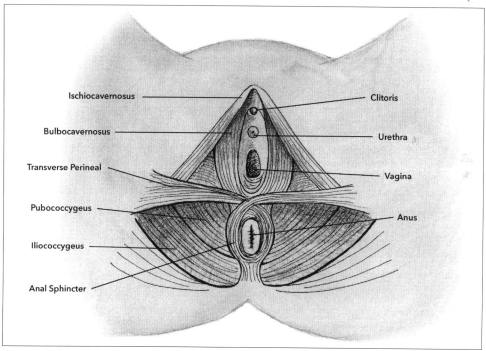

Figure 7. Superficial and Deep PFM (Vaginal View)

orectalis, and *iliococcygeus muscles.* The superficial layer is the *bulbocavernosus, ischiocavernosus, transverse perineal muscles* and the *anal sphincter muscle.*

The PFM are particularly critical to sexual function. The other core muscles and hip rotators are important with respect to the movements required for sex, but the PFM are unique as they directly involve the genitals. During arousal they help increase pelvic blood flow, contributing to vaginal lubrication, genital engorgement and the transformation of the clitoris from flaccid to softly swollen to rigid. The PFM enable the ability to tighten the vagina at will and compress the roots of the clitoris, elevating blood pressure within the clitoris to maintain clitoral erection. An orgasm would not be an orgasm without the contribution of PFM contractions.

WHO KNEW? *Pilates—emphasizing core strength, stability and flexibility—is a great source of PFM strength and endurance training. By increasing range of motion, loosening tight hips and spines and improving one's ability to rock and gyrate the hips, Pilates is an ideal exercise for improving sexual function.*

PFMT to Enhance Sexual Function: The Ultimate Sexercise

Note: The specifics of the PFMT program tailored for improving sexual function are covered in Chapter 13.

WHO KNEW? *The emerging concept of "vaginal health" has brought novel and at times questionable techniques into vogue. These include vaginal "steaming," vaginal "rejuvenation," vaginal "lasering," vaginal "sculpting" (using light, heat and sonic technology) and "vaginoplasty" surgery, etc. How about the classic, old school, low-tech, non-invasive Kegel PFMT as a starting point for vaginal fitness?*

Recall that the PFM have an intimate involvement with all aspects of sexuality from arousal to climax. They are highly responsive to sexual stimulation and react by contracting and increasing blood flow to the entire pelvic region, enhancing arousal. Upon clitoral stimulation, the PFM reflexively contract (via the BCR). When the PFM are voluntarily engaged, pelvic blood flow and sexual response are further intensified. During orgasm, the PFM contract involuntarily in a rhythmic fashion and provide the muscle power behind the physical aspect of an orgasm. The bottom line is that the pleasurable sensation that one perceives during sex is directly related to PFM function. Weakened PFM are clearly associated with sexual and orgasmic dysfunction.

PFMT improves PFM awareness, strength, endurance, tone and flexibility and can enhance sexual function in women with desire, arousal, orgasm and pain issues, as well as in women without sexual issues. PFMT helps sculpt a fit and firm vagina, which can positively influence sexual arousal and help one achieve an orgasm. PFMT results in increased muscle mass and more powerful PFM contractions and better PFM stamina, heightening the capacity for enhancing orgasm intensity and experiencing more orgasms as well as increasing "his" pleasure. PFMT is an excellent means of counteracting the adverse sexual effects of obstetrical trauma. Furthermore, PFMT can help prevent sexual problems that may emerge in the future.

WHO KNEW?   *A 2014 Norwegian study tested if PFMT could improve sexual function in women with POP. 40% of the women in the PFMT group noted improved sexual function vs. only 5% in a comparable group of women who did not pursue PFMT. Those in the PFMT group noted increased awareness, control and strength of the PFM. They also experienced the sensation of a tighter vagina, enhanced libido and orgasm, resolution of pain with sex, heightened partner satisfaction as well as more overall confidence.*

WHO KNEW?   *Strong PFM = Strong Orgasms. PFMT can lead to stronger and more satisfying orgasms. PFMT can revitalize the PFM and instill the capacity to activate the PFM with less effort. Over time, this can lead to enhanced muscle memory, more easily obtainable orgasms of greater intensity and the capacity to achieve multiple orgasms. Women capable of achieving "seismic" orgasms most often have very strong, toned, supple and flexible PFM.*

Tapping into and harnessing the energy of the PFM is capable of providing the erotic capital that translates into an improved sexual experience. If the core muscles are the "powerhouse" of the body, the PFM are the "powerhouse" of the vagina.

7 BLADDER WORKS

All leaky bladders cause urinary incontinence; however, all leaky bladders are not the same, as there are different underlying causes that require different treatments. The PFM are intimately involved with bladder support and function, contributing vitally to urinary control. This chapter is a brief overview of bladder anatomy and function to help you better understand the two most common forms of urinary leakage—stress urinary incontinence and overactive bladder— covered in the chapters that follow.

Bladder Control Issues—More Than Just a Physical Problem

Urinary incontinence is a condition in which one experiences involuntary leakage of urine. Although not life-threatening, it can be life-altering and life-disrupting. Many women resort to pads, living unhappily and uncomfortably with this debilitating, yet treatable problem. It is more than just a medical problem, often affecting emotional, psychological, social and financial well-being (the cumulative cost of pads can be significant). Many women are reluctant to participate in activities that provoke the incontinence, resulting in social isolation, loss of self-esteem and, at times, depression. Since exercise is a common trigger, many women avoid it, which can lead to weight gain and a decline in fitness. Sufferers often feel "imprisoned" by their bladders, which have taken control over their lives, impacting not only activities, but also clothing choices, travel plans and relationships.

Bladder Function 101

The *bladder* is a muscular balloon that has two functions, *storage* and *emptying* of urine. The stem of the bladder balloon is the *urethra*, the straw-like tube that conducts urine from the bladder during urination and helps store urine at all other times. The urethra runs from the *bladder neck* (where the urinary bladder and urethra join) to the *urethral*

Figure 8. Bladder

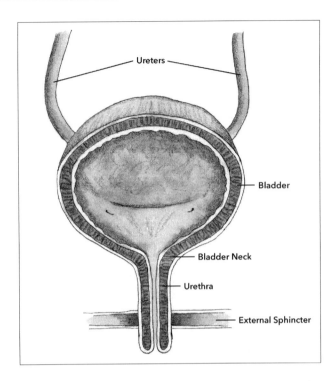

meatus, the external opening located just above the vagina on the vestibule. Healthy bladder functioning is contingent upon certain properties of the bladder and urethra. Bladder control issues arise when one or more of these go awry:

Capacity

The average adult has a bladder that holds about 12 ounces before a significant urge to urinate occurs. *Problem*: The capacity of the bladder is too small, giving rise to the frequent need to urinate.

Elasticity

The bladder is stretchy like a balloon and as it fills up there is a minimal increase in bladder pressure. Low-pressure storage is desirable, as the less pressure in the bladder, the less likelihood for leakage issues. *Problem*: The bladder is inelastic and stores urine at high pressures, a setup for urinary leakage.

Sensation

There is an increasing feeling of urgency as the urine volume in the bladder increases. *Problem*: There is heightened sensation creating a sense of urgency before the bladder is full, giving rise to the frequent need to urinate.

Contractility

After the bladder fills and the desire to urinate is sensed, a voluntary bladder contraction occurs, which increases the pressure within the bladder in order to generate the power to urinate. *Problem*: The bladder is "underactive" and cannot generate enough pressure to empty effectively, which may cause it to overflow when there are large volumes of urine that remain in the bladder.

Timing

A bladder contraction should only occur after the bladder is reasonably full. *Problem*: The bladder is "overactive" and squeezes prematurely (has an involuntary bladder contraction) causing a sudden urgency with the possibility of urinary leakage occurring en route to the bathroom.

Anatomical Position

The bladder and urethra are maintained in proper anatomical position in the pelvis because of PFM and connective tissue support. *Problem*: A weakened support system can cause urinary leakage with sudden increases in abdominal pressure, such as occurs with sneezing or coughing.

Urethra

In cross-section, the urethra has infoldings of its inner layer that give it a "snowflake-like" appearance. This inner layer is surrounded by rich, spongy tissue containing an abundance of blood vessels, creating a cushion around the urethra that permits a watertight seal similar to a washer in a sink. *Problem*: The female hormone *estrogen* nourishes the urethra; with declining levels of estrogen at the time of menopause, the urethra loses tone and suppleness, analogous to a washer in a sink becoming brittle, potentially causing leakage issues.

Sphincters

The urinary sphincters, located at the bladder neck and mid-urethra, are specialized muscles that provide urinary control by pinching the urethra closed during storage and allowing the urethra to open during emptying. The *main sphincter* is located at the bladder neck and is composed of smooth muscle designed for involuntary, sustained control. The *auxiliary sphincter* (a.k.a. the external sphincter), located further downstream and comprised of skeletal muscle contributed to by the PFM, is designed for voluntary, emergency control. *Problem*: Damage to or weakness of the sphincters adversely affects urinary control.

WHO KNEW?   *I liken the main sphincter to the brakes of a car—frequently used, efficient and effective. The auxiliary sphincter is similar to the emergency brake—much less frequently used, less efficient, but effective in a pinch. The PFM are intimately involved with the function of the "emergency brake."*

Nerves

The seemingly "simple" act of urination is actually a complex event requiring a functional nervous system that allows sensation of bladder filling and contraction of the bladder muscle along with the coordinated relaxation of the sphincters. *Problem*: Any neurological problem can adversely affect urination, causing bladder control issues.

Bladder Reflexes

A reflex is an automatic response to a stimulus, an action that occurs without conscious thought. There are three reflexes that are important to learn about since they are vital to bladder control.

Guarding Reflex: During bladder filling, the "guarding" PFM contract in increasing magnitude in proportion to the volume of urine in the bladder; this provides resistance that helps prevent leakage as the bladder becomes fuller.

Cough Reflex: With cough, there is a reflex contraction of the PFM, which helps prevent leakage with sudden increases in abdominal pressure.

Pelvic Floor Muscle-Bladder Reflex: When the PFM are voluntarily contracted, there is a reflex relaxation of the bladder. This powerful reflex can be tapped into for those who have involuntary bladder contractions that cause urgency and urgency leakage.

8

STRESS URINARY INCONTINENCE (SUI)

Tap into the powers of your PFM and harness the natural reflex that inhibits stress urinary incontinence.

Introduction

SUI is a very common condition that affects one in three women during their lifetimes, most often young or middle-aged women, although it can happen at any age. An involuntary spurt of urine occurs during sudden increases in abdominal pressure. This can happen with coughing, sneezing, laughing, jumping or exercise. It can even happen with walking, changing position from sitting to standing, or during sex.

In Europe, SUI is referred to as "exertion" incontinence, since some form of physical exertion usually triggers it. This is less confusing than the American term "stress" incontinence since the word stress has multiple meanings. In the context of SUI, stress means a sudden increase in abdominal pressure and not emotional tension.

WHO KNEW? *The triggers that most consistently induce SUI are vertical deceleration—jumping up with a sudden stop as one's feet touch down—typified by jumping jacks, using the trampoline and jumping rope.*

WHO KNEW? *There are hereditary/racial differences in the prevalence of SUI with SUI being less common in women of African descent and more common in Caucasian women, thought to be on the basis of genetic differences in the bulk of the PFM.*

Figure 9. Stress Urinary Incontinence

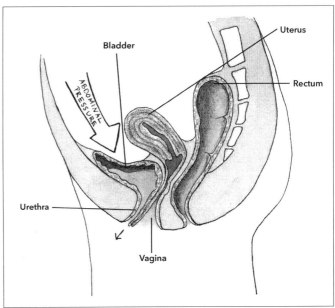

SUI most often occurs because the urethral support—PFM and connective tissues—has weakened and no longer provides an adequate "backboard" to the urethra. This allows the urethra to be pushed down and out of position at times of sudden increases in abdominal pressure, a condition known as *urethral hypermobility*. The foremost inciting factor for SUI is pregnancy, labor and delivery, particularly traumatic vaginal deliveries of large babies. SUI is uncommon in women who have not delivered a child vaginally or in women who have delivered by *elective* Caesarian section (a C-section without experiencing labor). However, *emergency* C-section when performed for failure of labor to progress confers a similar risk for SUI as does vaginal delivery.

Many women experience SUI during pregnancy. By their third month of pregnancy, 20% of women report SUI as do 50% at full term. There are many reasons for its occurrence, including the pressure of the enlarging uterus on the bladder and stretching of the PFM and other connective tissues.

WHO KNEW?   *After giving birth to your newborn, in addition to buying diapers for your baby you may have to buy them for yourself!*

WHO KNEW?   *The more vaginal deliveries one has, the greater the likelihood of developing SUI.*

WHO KNEW? *Numerous studies have demonstrated the benefits of post-partum PFMT in facilitating an early return of urinary control and improving the severity of SUI.*

Some women experience persistent SUI after childbirth, while others find that it improves dramatically and often resolves within 6 months. Others will not experience SUI until years after childbirth, after promoting factors have kicked in. These factors include obesity, aging, menopause, weight gain, gynecological surgery (especially hysterectomy), and any condition that increases abdominal pressure. These include coughing (often from smoking), asthma, weight training and high impact sports (e.g., trampoline, gymnastics, pole vaulting, etc.) and occupations that require heavy physical labor. Chronic constipation is a major contributory factor because of pushing and straining on a daily basis, cumulatively causing the same weakening of urethral support as happens with obstetrical labor.

WHO KNEW? *SUI is common in recreational as well as elite female athletes, particularly those who participate in high impact sports involving jumping. It can lead to poor athletic performance and ultimately avoiding participation in sports.*

The specific activities that provoke SUI and the severity of the leakage can vary greatly from woman to woman. Some only experience SUI with extreme exertion, such as with serving a tennis ball, swinging a golf club or with a powerful sneeze. Others experience SUI with minimal exertion such as walking or turning over in bed. Some women do not wear any protective pads or liners, changing their panties as necessary, whereas others wear many pads per day. Some are significantly bothered by even a minor degree of SUI, while others are accepting of experiencing many episodes of SUI daily.

Although the predominant cause of SUI is inadequate urethral support, it may also be caused by a weakened or damaged urethra itself. Risk factors for this are menopause, prior pelvic surgery, damage to the urethral nerve supply, radiation, and pelvic trauma. A severely compromised urethra usually causes significant urinary leakage with minimal activities and also results in "gravitational" incontinence, a profound urinary leakage that accompanies positional change.

Genuine SUI needs to be distinguished from other conditions that cause leakage of urine with increases in abdominal pressure that are *not* on the basis of inadequate urethral support or a weakened urethra. These other conditions can masquerade as genuine SUI. It is critical to distinguish between them since the treatments are very different. This is one reason why a thorough evaluation of SUI is important. The conditions that can masquerade as genuine SUI include the following: *failure to empty the bladder; urethral diverticulum; vaginal voiding;* and *stress-induced involuntary bladder contraction.*

Failure to empty the bladder can occur for a variety of reasons, including blockage of outflow of urine and an underactive bladder that contracts poorly. When the bladder is constantly full, it is easy to understand why a sudden increase in abdominal pressure can provoke leakage.

WHO KNEW? *An extension of this is that if your bladder is full and you leak a small amount with jumping or laughing, it is not necessarily problematic, but just means that you need to urinate before engaging in such activities.*

Urethral diverticulum is a small sac-like out-pouching from the urethra that can fill up with urine and leak during physical activities. The treatment is often surgical repair.

Vaginal voiding occurs in a small percentage of women who have an anatomical variation in which their urethral openings are somewhat internally recessed as opposed to the normal external urethral opening on the vestibule, immediately above the vaginal opening. When urinating, some of the urine pools in the vagina. Upon standing and physical exertion, the urine can then leak out of the vagina.

Stress-induced involuntary bladder contraction is a condition in which an involuntary contraction of the bladder is triggered by a maneuver that typically causes SUI. For example, a cough induces an involuntary bladder contraction, causing urinary leakage.

Diagnosis of SUI

SUI is on the spectrum of POP, since SUI is most often caused by weakened pelvic support. The diagnostic evaluation of SUI is essentially the same as that for POP. In the interest of avoiding redundancy, please refer to Chapter 5, *Diagnosis of POP* for information on this.

Management of SUI

There are a variety of treatment options for SUI, ranging from non-invasive strategies to surgery. There are no effective medications for SUI. A detailed discussion of surgery is beyond the scope of this book, but suffice it to say that if one does not have an adequate response to first-line, non-invasive, conservative measures, surgery becomes an appropriate consideration. But why not initially try a natural approach that is cost-effective, uses few resources and is free from side effects?

PFMT for SUI

Note: The specifics of the program tailored for SUI are covered in Chapter 13.

Combatting SUI demands that the PFM contract strongly, rapidly and ultimately, reflexively. The goal of PFMT is to increase PFM strength, power, endurance and coordination to improve the urethral support and closure mechanism. PFMT has the potential to improve or cure SUI in those who suffer with the problem and prevent it in those who do not have it.

Recall the *cough reflex*, the reflex contraction of the PFM—above and beyond their resting tone—when you cough. This squeezes the urethra closed to help prevent leakage. This is nature's way of protecting you from incontinence with a sudden increase in abdominal pressure, defending you from cough-related SUI. Nature is teaching us an important lesson: a contraction of the PFM will help prevent SUI. An extension of this principle is to exercise the PFM to amplify strength and power to allow earlier activation and a more robust contraction of the PFM.

PFMT is most effective in women with mild or mild-moderate SUI. Chances are that if your SUI is moderate-severe, PFMT will be less effective. However, if not cured, the SUI can be improved, and that might be sufficient. PFMT increases PFM bulk and thickness, including the auxiliary sphincter, reducing the number of SUI episodes. Additionally, PFMT improves urethral support at rest and with straining, diminishing the urethral hypermobility that is characteristic of SUI. It also permits earlier activation of the PFM when coughing, more rapid repeated PFM contractions and more durable PFM contractions between coughs. PFMT is equally effective for pre-menopausal and post-menopausal women with SUI. PFMT can cure or considerably improve 60-70% of women who suffer with SUI. The benefits persist for many years, as long as the exercises are adhered to on an ongoing basis.

Once you have achieved conditioned PFM via PFMT, it is vital to apply your improved PFM facility. You can replicate the cough reflex—voluntarily—when you are in situations other than actual coughing that induce SUI. In order to do so, you need to be attentive to the triggers that provoke your SUI. By actively contracting your PFM immediately prior to the trigger exposure, the SUI can be improved or prevented.

For example, if changing position from sitting to standing results in SUI, consciously performing a brisk PFM contraction—an intense contraction for 2-5 seconds prior to and during transitioning from sitting to standing—should "clamp the urethra" and help control the problem. Such bracing of the PFM can be a highly effective means of managing SUI and when practiced diligently can become automatic (a reflex behavior).

WHO KNEW? *A contemporary clinical study compared a large group of women pregnant with their first child, half of whom underwent a PFMT program and the other half of whom did not, concluding that PFMT was effective in the prevention of incontinence.*

Behavioral Advice: Additional Non-Invasive Strategies to Improve SUI

Manage the condition that provokes the SUI: Since discrete triggers often provoke SUI (e.g., when asthma causes wheezing, seasonal allergies cause sneezing, or when tobacco use, bronchitis, sinusitis, or postnasal drip cause coughing), by managing the underlying condition, the SUI can be avoided.

Moderate fluid intake: With a sudden increase in abdominal pressure, there will tend to be more SUI when there are larger volumes in the bladder (although SUI can occur even immediately after urinating). Since there is a direct relationship between fluid intake and urine production, any moderation in fluid intake will decrease the volume of urine in the bladder and potentially improve the SUI. The key is to find the right balance to diminish the SUI, yet avoid dehydration. Since caffeinated beverages and alcohol increase urine volume, it is best to limit exposure (caffeine is present in coffee, tea, cola and even chocolate has a caffeine-like ingredient).

Urinate regularly: Based on the premise that there tends to be more SUI when there are greater volumes in the bladder, by emptying your bladder more frequently, SUI can be better controlled. Urinating on a two-hour basis is usually effective, although the specific timetable needs to be individually tailored. *Voluntary* urinary frequency is more desirable than *involuntary* SUI. An extension of this principle is to empty your bladder immediately before any activity that is likely to induce the SUI.

Maintain a healthy weight: Extra pounds can worsen SUI by increasing abdominal pressure and placing a greater load on the pelvic floor and bladder. Even a modest weight loss may improve SUI.

WHO KNEW? *Bearing the burden of unnecessary pounds adversely affects many body parts. As much as obesity puts a great strain on the knees that support the body's weight, so it does on the PFM.*

Exercise: Being physically active can go a long way towards maintaining general fitness and helping improve SUI. In general, exercises that emphasize the core muscles—particularly Pilates and yoga—are most helpful for SUI. Unfortunately, and ironically, it is exercise that often provokes SUI.

WHO KNEW? *A Brazilian scientific study investigated the impact of physical activity on PFM strength, measured objectively via electromyography (EMG). Three populations of women were compared: a sedentary group; a group that walked; and a group that played volleyball regularly. The sedentary group had the weakest PFM strength, the walkers intermediate strength, and the volleyball players the greatest PFM strength. The authors concluded that higher impact sports force the PFM into greater activity.*

Tobacco cessation: Tobacco causes bronchial irritation and coughing that provoke SUI. Additionally, chemical constituents of tobacco constrict blood vessels, impair blood flow, decrease tissue oxygenation and promote inflammation, negatively affecting function of the bladder, urethra and PFM. By eliminating tobacco, SUI can be significantly improved.

Maintain bowel regularity: Achieving bowel regularity may improve SUI and prevent it from progressing. A rectum full of stool can adversely affect urinary control by putting internal pressure on the bladder and urethra. Additionally, chronic straining with bowel movements—similar in many ways to being in "labor" every day—can have a cumulative effect in weakening PFM and can be a key factor in the development of SUI. To promote healthy bowel function, exercise daily and increase your fiber intake by eating whole grains, fruits and vegetables.

The tampon trick: If SUI occurs under very predictable circumstances—e.g., during tennis, golf or jogging—a strategically placed tampon can be your friend. The tampon is not used for absorption purposes, but to support the urethra. By positioning the tampon in the vagina directly under the urethra, it acts as a space-occupying backboard. The tampon does not need to be positioned as deeply as it would be for menstruation, but just within the vagina. This may allow you to pursue your activities without the need for a pad. Caution: Be careful about leaving tampons in for prolonged times because of the risk of toxic shock syndrome. Poise has come out with "Impressa," a tampon available in three sizes designed specifically for SUI. It is placed via an applicator and can be worn for up to eight hours. In Australia and the UK, "Contiform," a self-inserted, foldable intra-vaginal device that is shaped like a hollow tampon, is often used to help manage SUI.

WHO KNEW? *If conservative measures fail to sufficiently improve your SUI, there are other solutions. A relatively simple outpatient procedure—the mid-urethral sling—is the implantation of a tape beneath the urethra to recreate the "backboard" of urethral support that is defective. The sling works to stabilize and provide hammock-like support to the urethra such that when a trigger of SUI occurs, the urethra will be compressed into the sling, which pinches the urethra closed.*

9 OVERACTIVE BLADDER (OAB) AND URGENCY URINARY INCONTINENCE (UUI)

Tap into the powers of your PFM and harness the natural reflex that inhibits urinary urgency, frequency and urgency incontinence.

Introduction

OAB is a common condition that can occur at any age, although it is more prevalent with aging. The key symptom of OAB is urinary urgency (a.k.a. "gotta go"), the sudden and compelling desire to urinate that is difficult to postpone. Other symptoms are urinating frequently during daytime and sleep time hours and urinary leakage (urgency urinary incontinence or UUI). It is often due to *involuntary bladder contractions* in which your bladder squeezes—suddenly and inappropriately so—without your "permission."

WHO KNEW? *Although UUI and SUI both result in leakage, there are many differences. With UUI, there is typically a large volume of urinary leakage, often associated with a strong urgency to urinate. With SUI, there is usually a small spurt of urinary leakage that occurs with very defined physical activities. Whereas UUI is due to involuntary bladder contractions, SUI is usually caused by weakened support of the urethra, or more rarely, a damaged urethra. SUI is somewhat predictable, UUI less so. Mixed incontinence is when both SUI and UUI coexist. With mixed incontinence it is prudent to initially manage the predominant type.*

Figure 10. Urgency Urinary Incontinence

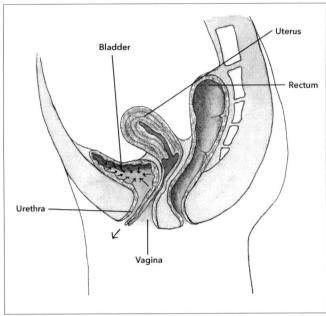

UUI can be the presenting symptom of a bladder irritation (e.g., a bladder infection or stone), obstruction (e.g., from a dropped bladder), or neurological disease (e.g., stroke, Parkinson's disease, multiple sclerosis, etc.).

Women with OAB typically urinate more than eight times daily and at least twice nightly, if not more. OAB can cause the feeling that one needs to urinate even though they just did. Despite one's best effort to hurry to the bathroom, urinary leakage often occurs. The sleep interruptions are particularly annoying, often causing daytime sleepiness. OAB can severely affect quality of life, causing constant disruptions to work and other activities and interfering with social activities, travel and sexual intimacy.

WHO KNEW?   *The bladder is a convenient outlet for stress and anxiety, which can be "channeled" to the bladder, causing symptoms of OAB.*

Ivan Pavlov (1849-1936) was a Russian physician, physiologist and psychologist who won the 1904 Nobel Prize in medicine. He is best known for describing *classical conditioning*. He exposed dogs to meat, which instinctually caused them to salivate—an "unconditioned response." He then used a bell to summon the dogs to a meaty meal and after a few cycles of repetition, the dogs began to salivate to just the sound of the bell. The reaction to the bell is called a "conditioned response," since it is a learned behavior. This is relevant to the human bladder, which is susceptible to such conditioning.

WHO KNEW?   *In an effort to teach young children to urinate on command, parents often seat them on the toilet and turn the faucet on, creating and reinforcing an association between running water and urinating. Unfortunately, many years later this conditioned response can trigger involuntary bladder contractions with exposure to running water, inducing urgency and perhaps UUI.*

Although UUI often occurs without provocation, it is commonly triggered by cues that are reminders of the act of emptying the bladder, generating a conditioned response (e.g., running faucets, approaching a bathroom, entering your home, etc.). "Latchkey" incontinence is a common condition in which placing the key in the door lock induces intense urgency and the need to scramble to get to the bathroom.

WHO KNEW?   *When I was a child I often had the sudden desire to urinate when I brushed my teeth. For years, I was perplexed, thinking it had something to do with dental hygiene, only to realize much later that it had nothing to do with the toothbrush, toothpaste or act of brushing, but with the running tap water ... yet another reason to shut off the water when you are brushing your teeth. Save the planet!*

WHO KNEW?   *In summer camp, we sometimes placed our sleeping bunkmate's hand in warm water to provoke him to wet the bed. It was all giggles for us and little did we know we were triggering a bladder contraction by way of a conditioned response.*

Diagnosis of OAB

A careful history, physical exam and urinalysis are often all that are necessary to diagnose OAB. A voiding diary—a 24-hour record of when you urinate and the volume of each urination—is a simple and helpful tool. In some patients, additional measures may be necessary to confirm the diagnosis, exclude other issues and help guide the treatment.

Depending upon circumstances, additional means to further evaluate OAB may include an endoscopic inspection of the lining of the bladder and urethra (cystoscopy), sophisticated functional tests of bladder storage and emptying (urodynamics) and, on occasion, imaging tests such as ultrasonography of the urinary tract.

Management of OAB

There are a variety of treatment options for OAB, ranging from non-invasive strategies to pills to surgery. A discussion of medications and surgery is beyond the scope of this book, but suffice it to say that if you do not have a satisfactory response to first-line, non-invasive, conservative measures, it would be appropriate to consider more aggressive treatments. But why not initially try the natural approach that costs nothing and is free from side effects?

PFMT for OAB and UUI

Note: The specifics of the PFMT program tailored for OAB/UUI are covered in Chapter 13.

During urine storage the bladder muscle is relaxed and the urinary sphincters are contracted; during urine emptying the bladder muscle contracts and the sphincter muscles relax. The actions of the bladder muscle and sphincter muscles are always in opposition—when the bladder is "on," the sphincters are "off," and when the bladder is "off," the sphincters are "on." This relationship can be used to your advantage if you suffer with OAB. Since those with OAB often have bladders that contract involuntarily, causing the symptoms of urgency, frequency and UUI, a means of relaxing the bladder is to intentionally engage the PFM to benefit from the reflex relaxation of the bladder that follows.

Recall that the PFM-bladder reflex is a *relaxation* of the bladder when you voluntarily contract the PFM. This reflex is unique because it results in the relaxation of a muscle as opposed to most reflexes, which result in muscle *contraction.* Deploying this reflex helps urinary urgency diminish or disappear and can effectively prevent or forestall urinary leakage. Numerous studies have demonstrated the benefits of PFMT for strengthening this reflex. In fact, the American Urological Association guidelines for OAB specify that PFMT is first-line therapy for OAB. The goal of PFMT is to increase PFM strength, power and endurance as well as to improve your capacity to inhibit involuntary bladder contractions. PFMT is one of the most effective remedies for combatting OAB by helping this inhibitory reflex to become more robust.

Once you have achieved PFM proficiency through PFMT, it becomes critical to apply this facility. To do so, when you feel the sudden and urgent desire to urinate, briefly but intensively pulse the PFM several times. When the PFM are rhythmically snapped in this manner, the bladder muscle reflexively relaxes and the feeling of intense urgency should disappear.

WHO KNEW?   *Using this reflex to your advantage is a keeper when you are stuck in traffic and have no access to a toilet, regardless if you have OAB or not. Note that if your bladder is filled to capacity, the relief of the urinary urgency will be short lived.*

Going beyond inhibiting the problem *after* it occurs is *preventing* it from occurring in the first place. In order to do so, it is important to recognize the specific triggers that induce your urgency, frequency or UUI: hand washing, key in the door, rising from sitting, running water, entering the shower, cold or rainy weather, etc. Prior to trigger exposure, "snapping" the PFM rapidly several times can preempt the abnormal bladder contraction before it occurs.

Behavioral Advice: Additional Non-Invasive Strategies to Improve OAB

The most effective non-invasive treatment of OAB is a combination of PFMT with behavioral modifications.

Moderate fluid intake and avoid bladder irritants: The intake of large volumes of fluids and certain beverages, particularly those that can irritate the bladder—including alcohol and caffeine (coffee, tea, cola and chocolate)—can worsen symptoms of OAB. There is a prevalent misconception that 8-10 glasses of water per day are necessary for good health. Although water is vital for many body functions and to prevent dehydration, it is advisable to drink in accordance with your thirst just as you would sleep in accordance with your fatigue level. Any restriction in fluid intake will decrease the volume of urine. Since urgency and UUI often do not occur until a "critical" urinary volume is reached, by curbing fluid intake it will take a longer time to reach this critical volume. The key is to find the right balance to improve control but avoid dehydration. Additional bladder irritants include carbonated beverages, artificial sweeteners, citrus products, tomatoes and tomato products and spicy foods. If you find that any of these worsen your OAB symptoms, it would be advisable to minimize your intake of them.

Urinate regularly: For UUI, urinating on a schedule and not by your own sense of urgency will keep your bladder as empty as possible. By emptying your bladder before the "critical" volume is reached, urinary leakage can be controlled. Urinating on a two-hour basis is usually effective, although the specific timetable has to be tailored to the individual. Such "preemptive" urinating has proven to be a useful technique since *voluntary* urinary frequency is more desirable than *involuntary* leakage. Remember to urinate immediately prior to sleeping. "Double" voiding—emptying your bladder as completely as possible and then attempting to urinate a second time—can be helpful for those who have difficulty emptying their bladders completely.

Bladder retraining: This is appropriate for those who have urgency and frequency without UUI. Bladder retraining involves gradually increasing the interval between urinating to establish normal voiding patterns. The premise is that your sense of urgency is not a reliable measure of the status of your bladder filling, as the urgency often occurs with small bladder volumes. Urinating by the "clock" and not by your sense of urgency will help normalize your urinary volumes. Urinating on a two-hour basis is usually effective as a starting point, although the specific timetable has to be tailored, based upon how often you actually urinate. A gradual and progressive increase in the interval between urinating can be achieved by consciously delaying urinating. A goal of an increase in the voiding interval by 15-30 minutes per week is desirable and eventually a return to more acceptable intervals of urinating every four hours or so is possible. Reacting to the initial sense of urgency by running to the bathroom needs to be replaced with urgency inhibition techniques: Stop in your tracks, sit, breathe deeply, relax and pulse your PFM rhythmically to resist and suppress urgency.

Maintain a healthy weight: Extra pounds can worsen OAB issues by putting pressure on the urinary bladder. Even a modest weight loss may improve OAB symptoms.

Exercise: Physical activities can help maintain general fitness and improve urinary control issues. In general, lower impact exercises—yoga, Pilates, cycling, swimming, etc.—can best help alleviate pressure on the urinary bladder by boosting core muscle strength and tone and improving posture and alignment.

Tobacco cessation: The chemical constituents of tobacco constrict blood vessels, impair blood flow, decrease tissue oxygenation and promote inflammation, compromising the bladder, urethra and PFM. By eliminating tobacco, symptoms of OAB can be improved.

Maintain bowel regularity: A full rectum can create internal pressure on the urinary bladder and provoke urinary urgency, similar to how externally pushing on the lower abdomen can induce the urge to urinate. Bowel regularity may thus be of aid in improving OAB. To promote healthy bowel function, exercise daily and increase fiber intake.

WHO KNEW? *If conservative measures—including PFMT—fail to sufficiently improve OAB symptoms, there are other solutions. There are numerous oral medications of several different classes that can* *improve or cure the symptoms of OAB by relaxing the bladder muscle. Botox (Botulinum toxin) injections into the bladder can substantially enhance the quality of life of women suffering with OAB by causing temporary paralysis of segments of the bladder muscle. Sacral neuro-modulation delivers electrical pulses to nerves that affect bladder function, reducing the symptoms of OAB. One form of neuro-modulation is percutaneous tibial nerve stimulation, in which a needle is inserted near the tibial nerve in the ankle and a hand-held stimulator generates electrical stimulation. Another form of sacral neuro-modulation is the insertion of a permanent bladder "pacemaker" that provides battery-powered electrical impulses to the sacral nerves that affect bladder function.*

10 A FEW WORDS ON BOWEL CONTROL AND THE PFM

The bladder and the bowel share much in common. Just as PFMT can improve SUI and OAB, so it can improve bowel control issues including bowel urgency and bowel incontinence.

The urinary and intestinal tracts have many similarities. They are geographical next-door neighbors, have essentially the same nerve supply, and travel from the pelvis to the perineum via openings in the PFM. The PFM play a vital role in the anatomical support and control functions of both tracts and contribute to the anal sphincter just as they do to the urethral sphincter. The bladder and rectum share the same inhibitory reflex in which a voluntary contraction of the PFM results in relaxation.

Bowel incontinence is a dreadful and embarrassing problem in which there is accidental leakage of rectal contents. It can be due to involuntary rectal contractions, an impaired anal sphincter, or situational issues such as diarrhea, being on a bowel "prep" for a colonoscopy, or lack of access to a toilet.

As beneficial as snapping the PFM are for suppressing involuntary bladder contractions, so they have equal use for suppressing involuntary bowel contractions that can cause bowel urgency and incontinence. At the time of the perceived bowel urgency, rhythmic pulsing of the PFM can diminish or abort the involuntary bowel contraction. PFMT helps stimulate the inhibitory reflex between the PFM and the bowel muscle and as the inhibitory reflex becomes more robust, you develop an enhanced ability to counteract bowel urgency and urgency incontinence.

PFMT can also help improve bowel incontinence for those suffering with anal sphincter impairments. Since the anal sphincter is part of the

PFM, a conditioning program will increase its strength, tone and power as well as the capacity for a voluntary, sustained and powerful contraction of the anal sphincter.

Note: The specifics of the PFMT program tailored for bowel urgency/incontinence are covered in Chapter 13.

11 PELVIC PAIN CAUSED BY PFM TENSION MYALGIA

Entire books are devoted to the complex topic of female pelvic pain, which afflicts about 30 million women in the U.S. Pelvic pain has numerous causes with PFM dysfunction being a common component. This brief chapter covers pelvic pain caused by a type of PFM dysfunction in which the PFM are over-tensioned, a condition that can be improved by learning how to relax the PFM.

Introduction

Any muscle in the body can be afflicted with tension issues, and the PFM are no exception. "Tension myalgia" of the PFM—tightness, spasticity and inflammation due to the PFM being in a state of hyper-contraction—is a not uncommon condition that can cause intense pelvic pain and other symptoms. It is a very difficult and frustrating situation that requires a number of different treatment approaches.

WHO KNEW? *Tension myalgia of the PFM can create the sensation that one's PFM are "tied in a knot." There exist actual PFM "knots," also known as "myofascial trigger points," which are discrete sites of hyper-tensioned muscle.*

In this condition, one or more of the pelvic muscles exists in an over-contracted state. Because the pelvis is home to urinary, sexual and bowel function, it is a particularly bad location for holding tension. PFM "hypertension" can give rise to urinary, genital and rectal pain as well as adversely affect the function of these systems. PFM tension myalgia can cause difficulty starting one's urinary stream, a weak stream, incomplete emptying of the bladder and overactive bladder symptoms. It can give rise to pain with sexual stimulation and intercourse, sometimes to the extent that sexual intercourse is not possible. It can also cause constipation, hemorrhoids, fissures and other bowel symptoms.

This "headache" of the PFM is often provoked by anxiety and stress. It is theorized that this chronically over-contracted group of muscles is a manifestation of stress turned inwards, a subconscious response to stress and a classic example of the mind-body connection. From a psychological perspective, this state of "chronic hyper-vigilance" of the PFM seemingly serves the purpose of guarding and protecting the genital and anal areas. When anxiety expresses itself through tension in the PFM, the physical tension and pain further contribute to emotional anxiety and a stress reaction, which creates a vicious cycle. Poor posture, muscle overuse and an abnormality with the nerve pathway that regulates muscle tone are other factors that are thought to contribute to tension myalgia.

WHO KNEW?   *In many ways, PFM tension myalgia is similar to tension headaches, a not uncommon response to stress.*

WHO KNEW?   *PFM tension myalgia parallels what a frightened dog does when it pulls its tail between its legs, hyper-contracting its PFM in an effort to protect a vulnerable region of its body.*

Characteristically, the pain waxes and wanes in intensity over time, wanders to different locations and can be perceived to be superficial, intermediate or deep in the pelvis. It can involve the lower abdomen, groin, pubic area, clitoris, labia, vagina, perineum, anus, rectum, hips and lower back. The pain is often described as "stabbing," although it can be cramping, burning or itching in quality. Urination, bowel movements, sexual activity or wearing tight clothing can aggravate the pain.

Because the symptoms of tension myalgia of the PFM can be vague and variable, afflicted women often have difficulty expressing their symptoms in a precise way, although they usually have a long list of issues, have typically seen many physicians and have had numerous prior interventions. Many patients thought to have *interstitial cystitis/chronic pelvic pain syndrome, irritable bowel syndrome, vulvodynia* or *fibromyalgia* in actuality have tension myalgia of the PFM. In fact, PFM tension myalgia is probably one of the most common problems that urologists and gynecologists see and is likely one of the most misunderstood, misdiagnosed and mistreated conditions. Many suffering with PFM tension myalgia are miserable and deeply frustrated because of having endured years of episodic agony without relief.

WHO KNEW?   *Sufferers often describe the sensation of a foreign object in the vagina, likely because of the bulkiness of the PFM in the chronically contracted state.*

Diagnosis of PFM Tension Myalgia

After having identified PFM tension myalgia in many patients, in retrospect it seems to have been such an obvious diagnosis. A careful history and a physical exam can usually establish this diagnosis. Most important is a pelvic exam to evaluate the superficial and deep PFM. Typical findings are tight and tender PFM, spasticity, difficulty in relaxing the PFM following contraction and weak PFM strength. Localized, knot-like bands can often be felt within the PFM, similar to tension knots that can develop in back muscles. The pain can often be localized by a vaginal or rectal exam that identifies these trigger points, the sites of origin of the myalgia that when manipulated cause tremendous pain, often replicating the symptoms. The jury is not out on why these trigger points cause discomfort and pain. One school of thought is diminished blood flow to these specific areas and an alternative theory is that the pain is neurological, brought on by inflamed nerve endings.

Unfortunately, conventional urology and gynecology medical practices are more nuts-and-bolts and mechanistic than psychological in orientation and have been slow to embrace the concept that stress and other psychosocial factors can give rise to physical complaints. As such, PFM tension myalgia is often not even considered as a possible diagnosis. However, an understanding of this condition is slowly gaining recognition and traction.

Management of PFM Tension Myalgia

The key to treating PFM tension myalgia is to foster relaxation and "down-training" of the spastic PFM in order to untie the "knot(s)." By making the proper diagnosis and providing pain relief, the vicious cycle of anxiety/pain can be broken. Managing PFM tension myalgia often requires multiple approaches including anti-inflammatory and anti-spasmodic medications, stress management and focused therapies including application of heat and pelvic massage. Pelvic floor physical therapists use a number of physical interventions that provide PFM stretching and lengthening to increase the flexibility of the PFM, including trigger point therapy, which involves compressing and massaging the knotted and spastic muscles.

WHO KNEW?   *Those afflicted with PFM tension myalgia who are so motivated can pursue self-treatment regimens using internal, manually guided trigger point release wands that aim to relieve or eliminate the knots by self-directed manipulation and massage. These devices may be obtained without a prescription and are available online.*

PFMT can be a useful piece of this multimodal management approach by its focus on developing proficiency in *relaxing* the PFM. The emphasis here is not on *contracting* these already over-contracted and over-tensioned muscles, which could aggravate the problem. This demands a different spin on the usual concept of PFMT, which in this instance is not to increase the tone and strength of the PFM—rather it is to instill PFM awareness and to enable the capacity for maximal PFM relaxation, which is considered to be a "meditative" state between PFM muscle contractions.

WHO KNEW?   *The relaxing aspect of PFMT is as important a component as is the contracting phase and is the key to managing PFM tension myalgia. Those suffering with this problem need to learn to unclench and release the PFM.*

WHO KNEW?   *PFM tension myalgia often demands multiple approaches. It sometimes requires injecting a medication—including anesthetics, steroids or Botox—into the offending trigger points.*

Note: The specifics of the PFMT program tailored for pelvic floor tension myalgia are covered in Chapter 13.

Note: Chapters 5-11 address those specific PFM dysfunctions that PFMT can benefit. Chapters 12-14 spell out the details of the various PFMT programs.

12 GETTING READY TO START PFMT

This chapter provides information on the fast twitch and slow twitch muscle fibers that determine PFM function, the adaptation principle, the distinction between strength, power and stability, the process of building muscle memory, how to develop PFM awareness and execute a proper PFM contraction and the means to assess your PFM strength and stamina.

Skeletal Muscle

Muscles are specialized tissues composed of *fibers* that contract (shorten and tighten) and relax (lengthen and loosen). Muscles provide shape to our bodies and allow for movement, stability and maintenance of posture. Most skeletal muscles come in pairs and cross bony joints—when one group contracts, it causes bending of that joint and when the opposing group contracts, it causes straightening of that joint (e.g., biceps/triceps). When each contracts equally, the joint will be in a neutral position. The human body has three types of muscles—*skeletal muscles* that provide mobility and stability, *smooth muscles* that line the arteries, bladder, intestine, etc., and the unique *cardiac muscle* of the heart.

The PFM are skeletal muscles comprised of both *fast twitch* and *slow twitch* muscle fibers. Fast twitch fibers predominate in high contractile muscles that fatigue rapidly and are used for fast-paced muscle action, e.g., sprinting. Slow twitch fibers predominate in endurance muscles, e.g., marathon running. The PFM have a baseline tone because of the presence of slow twitch fibers. The presence of fast twitch fibers allows their capacity for voluntary contraction. The PFM fibers are 70% slow twitch, fatigue-resistant, endurance muscles to maintain constant muscle tone (e.g., sphincter function and pelvic support) and 30% fast twitch, capable of rapid and powerful contractions (e.g., orgasm, interrupting your urinary stream and tightening your anus).

WHO KNEW? *Aging causes a decline in the function of the fast twitch fibers, but tends to spare the slow twitch fibers.*

Muscle mass is dynamic, a balance between growth and breakdown. As we age, muscle fiber wasting occurs as muscle breakdown exceeds muscle growth, which adversely affects function. Strength training is capable of reducing muscle wasting by increasing muscle bulk through enlargement of muscle fibers.

Adaptation

Exercise is about *adaptation*. Our muscles are remarkably adaptable to the stresses placed upon them and muscle growth will only occur in the presence of progressive overload, which causes compensatory structural and functional changes. That is why exercises get progressively easier in proportion to the effort put into doing them. As muscles adapt to the stresses placed upon them, a "new normal" level of fitness is achieved. Another term for adaptation is *plasticity*. Our muscles are "plastic," meaning they are capable of growth or shrinkage depending on the environment to which they are exposed.

The PFM are the same as other skeletal muscles in terms of their response to exercise. In accordance with the adaptation principle, it is advisable to increase repetitions and intensity in order to build muscle strength, power and endurance. As much as our muscles adapt positively to resistance, so they will adapt to the absence of stresses and resistance, resulting in smaller, weaker and less durable muscles.

WHO KNEW? *Use It or Lose It. With a conditioning regimen the PFM will thrive, optimizing their function. When the PFM are neglected, they will weaken, impairing their function.*

Strength, Power and Stability

The goal of PFM training is to maximize PFM *strength*, *power* and *stability*. *Strength* is the maximum amount of force that a muscle can exert. With time and effort, PFM contractions become more robust, helping sexual function and improving your ability to neutralize SUI, OAB and POP. *Power* is a gauge of strength and speed (muscle force multiplied by the contraction speed), a measure of how rapidly strength can be expressed, of great benefit to sexual health and the ability to react rapidly to urinary/bowel urgency and SUI. *Stability* helps maintain vaginal tone, urinary and bowel sphincter function and pelvic organ support as well as contributing to the "backboard" that helps prevent SUI.

Building Muscle Memory

It is important to understand how one becomes adept at using their muscles. This is relevant to gaining competence in *any* new physical activity and will be applied specifically to acquiring the skills to perform well-executed PFM contractions.

There are four stages of motor learning. (I learned this as it pertained to the mechanics of a golf swing, but it is equally relevant to mastering contracting the PFM.)

1. *Unconscious/incompetence*

There is no awareness of the motion and it cannot be capably performed. It is challenging to make the connection between your brain and your PFM because the PFM under most circumstances are used involuntarily without conscious awareness. This connection is not intuitive and must be taught.

WHO KNEW?   *The connections between your brain and PFM consist of sensory and motor nerves. The PFM contain sensors known as "proprioceptors" that detect stretch, position and motion and convey this information to the brain via sensory nerves. Motor nerves originate in the brain and enable the PFM to contract.*

2. *Conscious/incompetence*

Awareness of the motion is taught, but the motion cannot be competently performed.

3. *Conscious/competence*

Awareness of the motion is established and with sufficient practice the motion can be competently performed.

4. *Unconscious/competence*

With continued practice, the brain-PFM connection and muscle memory become well established and the motion can be performed reflexively without conscious thought or effort.

PFM Education and Awareness

Studies have shown that the majority of women with pelvic floor dysfunction referred for PFMT are unable to perform a proper voluntary PFM contraction and almost all demonstrate weak PFM strength regardless of age, nationality or diagnosis.

For years, physical therapists and physical medicine and rehabilitation experts have used *functional restoration* to effectively manage injured skeletal muscles. This strategy can likewise be applied to weakened and poorly functional PFM. The principles involve *segregation*, *guidance* and *progression*. Segregation is a thorough awareness of PFM anatomy and function as well as isolation of the PFM by contracting them independently of other muscles. Guidance refers to the directions and instructions necessary to learn how to properly engage and train the PFM. Progression refers to the incrementally more challenging exercises over the course of the PFMT regimen that result in PFM growth and improvement. Exercise is about adaptation, so increasing repetitions and intensity is mandatory to achieve results. The goal is for fit PFM—strong yet flexible PFM, equally capable of powerful contractions as well as full relaxation.

Initially, one must become aware and mindful of the presence, location and nature of the PFM. A good starting point is what the PFM are *not*: the PFM are not the muscles of the abdomen, thighs or buttocks, but are the saddle of muscles that run from the pubic bone in front to the tailbone in back.

The PFM have a resting tone, even though you are not typically aware of it. They can be contracted and relaxed at will: a voluntary contraction of the PFM will enable interruption of the urinary stream and tightening of the anal canal and an involuntary (reflex) contraction of the PFM occurs, for example, at the time of a cough. Relaxation of the PFM occurs during urination or a bowel movement.

Dr. Arnold Kegel described a PFM contraction as "a squeeze around the pelvic opening with an inward lift." With a proper PFM contraction, your perineum (the area between the vagina and anus) pulls in and lifts in an upward direction—"drawing in and up"—the very opposite feeling of "bearing down" to move your bowels. One method of getting the feel for doing a proper PFM contraction is to initially tighten the vagina and secondly the anus and then lift up the perineum.

WHO KNEW? *Kay Crotty, a prominent pelvic floor physiotherapist in the UK, found that it is initially easier to learn how to contract your PFM by concentrating on just the back PFM (anal sphincter). She also discovered that women who tighten their PFM while focused on both the front PFM (vaginal) and back PFM do better quality PFM contractions than those who tighten their PFM focused on just the front PFM.*

There are a number of mental images that can be useful in understanding PFM contractions. One is to think of the pubic bone and tailbone moving towards each other. Another helpful picture is to imagine the PFM as an elevator—when the PFM are engaged, the elevator rises upwards to the first floor from the ground floor; with continued training, the elevator rises to the second floor. Alternatively, envision that you are lifting a ping pong ball with your vagina and pulling it deep inside you. Another means is to mentally visualize that you are removing a tampon from your vagina and as you pull on the string you try to resist and hold the tampon in.

There are simple "biofeedback" techniques that can be helpful as well. After emptying your bladder about halfway, try to interrupt your urinary stream for a few seconds while you focus on the PFM that allow you to do so. Then resume and complete urination. The feeling should be that of clenching and unclenching the vagina, urethra and anus. Another method is to introduce a finger in your vagina and contract your PFM: the feeling should be of your vagina having a firm grip around your finger.

Doing It Right

PFM exercises must be done properly to reap the benefits that can be attained. Many women think they are doing these exercises correctly, but are found on examination to be contracting the wrong muscles, an explanation of why their efforts may have failed to improve their situation. To reiterate, PFM exercises involve pulling inwards and upwards, lifting and elevating and thereby tightening the urethral, vaginal and anal openings—the very opposite of straining. One strains to move their bowels, whereas one "Kegels" to accomplish the opposite—to tighten up the sphincters to NOT move their bowels; in fact, PFM contractions are a means of suppressing bowel urgency.

How do you know if you are contracting your PFM properly? It is helpful to use a hand-held mirror to look at your vaginal and anal regions in order to see what is happening when you contract your PFM.

Six Ways to Know That You Are Properly Contracting Your PFM

1. When you see the base of your clitoris retract and move inwards towards your pubic bone.

2. When you see your perineum (area between vagina and anus) move up and in.

3. When you see the anus contract ("anal wink") and feel the anus tighten and pull up and in.

4. When you can stop your urinary stream completely.

5. When you place your index and middle fingers on your perineum and you feel the contraction.

6. When you place a finger in your vagina, you feel the vaginal "grip" tighten.

WHO KNEW? *Vince Lombardi stated: "Practice doesn't make perfect, perfect practice makes perfect." This is wholly applicable to PFMT.*

Assessing Your PFM

There are many fancy ways of testing your PFM, but the simplest is by using tools that everyone owns—their fingers. *Digital palpation* (a finger in the vagina) is the standard means of testing the contraction strength of the PFM. The other methods are visual inspection, electromyography (electrical activity of the PFM), perineometry (measuring PFM contractile strength via a device that is inserted into the vagina) and imaging tests that assess the lifting aspects of the PFM, such as ultrasound and magnetic resonance imaging.

Assessment of your PFM evaluates your PFM strength and endurance. PFM strength can be self-assessed in the supine position (lying down, face up) with your knees bent and parted. Gently place a lubricated finger of one hand in the vagina and contract your PFM, lifting upwards and inwards and squeezing around the finger. Keep your buttocks down in contact with the surface you are lying on. Ensure that you are not contracting your gluteal (butt), rectus (abdomen) or adductor (inner thigh) muscles. Do this by placing your other hand on each of these other muscle groups, in turn, to prove to yourself that these muscles remain relaxed during the PFM contraction.

Rate your PFM strength using the modified *Oxford grading scale*, **giving yourself a grade ranging from 0-5.** Note that the Oxford system is what many physicians use and it is relatively simple when done regularly by those who are experienced performing pelvic exams. It is granted that since this is not your area of expertise, you may find this challenging. However, do your best to get a general sense of your baseline PFM strength.

Oxford Grading of PFM Strength

0   complete lack of contraction

1   minor flicker

2   weak squeeze (without a circular contraction or inner and upward movement)

3   moderate squeeze (with some inner and upward movement)

4   good squeeze (with moderate inner and upward movement)

5   strong squeeze (with significant inner and upward movement)

Next test your PFM endurance. Do as many PFM contractions as possible, pulsing the PFM rapidly until fatigue sets in (the failure point where you cannot do any more contractions). After you have recovered, contract the PFM for several seconds followed by relaxing them for several seconds, doing as many repetitions until fatigue occurs. Finally, do a single PFM contraction and hold it for as long as you can.

Record your Oxford grade and the maximum number of pulses, maximum number of several second contractions and the duration of sustained hold as baseline measurements. These will be useful to help assess your progress. Initially, it is likely that your PFM will be weak and lack endurance capacity.

13 BASIC PFMT PROGRAMS

Finally ... the nuts and bolts of PFMT! My interest and expertise in this area dates back to my fellowship training at UCLA in female pelvic medicine and reconstructive surgery, coupled with my passion for health, wellness and fitness. After decades in the urology/gynecology "trenches," I have concluded that PFMT is a vastly unexploited resource that offers significant benefits, yet comprehensive PFMT programs are few and far between.

"Strength training improves muscle vitality and function." These seven words embody a key principle of exercise physiology that is applicable to every muscle in the body, including the PFM.

Introduction

In terms of PFMT programs, there is no consensus regarding the following: the best position in which to do PFM exercises; the precise number of sets to perform daily; the number of repetitions per set; the intensity of PFM contractions; the duration of PFM contractions; the duration of PFM relaxation; and how often to do PFMT. The particulars of many PFMT routines are arbitrary at best. In fact, Campbell's Urology—the premier urology textbook—concludes: "No PFMT regimen has been proven most effective and treatment should be based on the exercise physiology literature."

My goal is to take the arbitrary out of PFMT, providing you with thoughtfully designed, specifically tailored programs crafted in accordance with Dr. Kegel's precepts, exercise physiology principles and practical concepts.

Dr. Kegel's precepts are summarized as follows (See Chapter 3 to review the details):

- Muscle education
- Feedback
- Progressive intensity
- Resistance

Exercise physiology principles as applied to PFMT include the following (note that there is some overlap with Dr. Kegel's precepts and practical concepts):

- Adaptation: The process by which muscle growth occurs in response to the demands placed upon the PFM, with adaptive change in proportion to the effort put into the exercises.

- Progression: The necessity for more challenging exercises in order to continue the process of adaptive change that occurs as "new normal" levels of PFM fitness are established. This translates into slowly and gradually increasing contraction intensity, duration of contractions, number of PFM repetitions and number of sets.

- Distinguishing strength, power and endurance training: Strength is the maximum amount of force that a muscle can exert; power is a measure of this strength factoring in speed, i.e., a measure of how quickly strength can be expressed. Endurance or stamina is the ability to sustain a PFM contraction for a prolonged time and the ability to perform multiple contractions before fatigue sets in. High intensity PFM contractions build muscle strength, whereas less intensive but more sustained contractions build endurance. Power is fostered by rapidly and explosively contracting the PFM.

- "Use it or lose it": The "plasticity" of the PFM—the adaptation in response to the specific demands placed on the muscles—requires continued training, at minimum a "maintenance" program after completion of a course of PFMT.

- Full range of motion: The goal of PFMT is not only to increase strength, power and endurance, but also flexibility. This is accomplished by bringing the muscle through the full range of motion, which at one extreme is full contraction (muscle shortening), and at the other, complete relaxation (muscle lengthening). The exception to this is for muscles that are already over-tensioned, which need to be relaxed through muscle lengthening exercises.

Practical concepts encompass the following:

- Initially training the PFM in positions that remove gravity from the picture, then advancing to positions that incorporate gravity.

- Beginning with the simplest, easiest, briefest PFM contractions, then proceeding with the more challenging, longer duration contractions.

- Slowly and gradually increasing exercise intensity and degree of difficulty.

- Aligning the specific pelvic floor dysfunction with the appropriate training program that focuses on improving the area of weakness, since each pelvic floor dysfunction is associated with specific deficits in strength, power and/or endurance.

The basic PFMT programs that follow are "low tech" exercises of the PFM without added resistance. They can be thought of as PFMT 101, which will provide the foundation for pelvic muscle proficiency. After mastery of basic PFMT, you can then progress to the next phase of conditioning—resistance training (the subject of the following chapter).

PFMT is the essence of "functional fitness," exercises that develop PFM strength, power, stamina and the skillset that can be used to improve and/or prevent specific functional impairments. PFMT regimens need to be flexible and nuanced, designed and customized with particular functional needs in mind, i.e., issues of prolapse, incontinence, sexual dysfunction, pain, etc., as opposed to a one-size-fits-all approach. An additional consideration is baseline PFM strength and stamina (as determined by the Oxford scale and endurance evaluation). After recognizing an area of weakness, focused effort should be applied to this deficit.

Time To Begin

At this point, you should have sufficient familiarity with your PFM to get started with basic PFMT. You do not need to go to a gym, wear athletic clothing, have any special equipment, or dedicate a great deal of time to this. It is vital to perform *quality* PFM contractions with the goal of slow and steady progress. Do not be surprised if you experience some aching and soreness as you begin PFMT.

If you are pursuing PFMT for specific pelvic issues, expect that it may take a number of weeks or more to see an improvement in your symptoms. After you have noticed a beneficial effect, the exercise regimen must be maintained, because regression can occur if the muscles are not consistently exercised.

Basic PFMT exercises can be performed lying down, sitting upright in a comfortable chair with your back straight, or standing. It is best to begin lying down, to minimize the element of gravity, which makes the exercises more challenging. Regardless of position, it is essential to maintain good form, posture and body alignment while doing PFMT. It is important to relax your abdomen, buttocks and thighs. Breathe slowly and do not hold your breath. Even though no muscle group works alone, by trying to *isolate* the PFM and focusing on squeezing only the PFM, you will make more rapid progress. You should not be grimacing, grunting or sweating, as PFMT is, in part, a meditative pursuit that employs awareness, focus, mindfulness and intention while performing deliberate contractions of the PFM.

WHO KNEW? *"Snap" effectively describes a brief, vigorous, energetic, well-executed contraction of the PFM. With increasing command of the PFM, they can be "snapped" like your fingers or the shutter of a camera.*

There are six variables with respect to PFMT: **contraction intensity; contraction duration; relaxation duration; power; repetitions;** and **number of sets** performed. Contraction intensity refers to the extent that the muscles are squeezed, ranging from a weak flick of the muscles to a robust and vigorous contraction. The contraction duration is the amount of time that the squeeze is sustained, ranging from a "snap"— a rapid pulsing of the PFM, to a "sustained hold"—a long duration contraction. The relaxation duration is the amount of time the PFM are unclenched until the next contraction is performed. Power is a measure of contraction strength and speed, the ability to rapidly achieve a full intensity contraction. Repetitions (reps) are the number of contractions performed in a single set (one unit of exercise).

It is relatively easy to intensively contract your PFM for a brief period, but difficult to maintain that intensity for a longer duration contraction. It is unlikely that you will be able to maintain the intensity of contraction of a sustained hold as you would for a snap.

PFMT regimens utilize snaps, few-second contractions and sustained duration contractions to reap the benefits of both strength and endurance training. The short duration, high intensity contractions will build strength and power and the longer duration, less intense contractions will build muscle endurance, both vital elements of fit PFM. Incremental change—the gradual and progressive increase in the intensity of contraction, duration of contraction, number of reps and number of sets performed—is the goal. Performing the PFMT programs 3-4 times weekly is desirable since recovery days are important for skeletal muscles.

PFMT is not an extreme program; nonetheless, it is by no means an undemanding program, requiring effort and perseverance. Depending on your level of baseline PFM fitness, you may find the exercises anywhere in the range from relatively easy to quite challenging. Your PFM are unique in terms of their shape, size and strength and consequently expectations regarding results will vary from individual to individual.

After one month, you should be on your way to achieving basic conditioning of the PFM. Reassessing the PFM by repeating the Oxford grading and the PFM endurance tests that you measured at baseline should demonstrate *objective* evidence of progress. More importantly, you should start noticing *subjective* improvement in many of the domains that PFM fitness can influence. Once you have mastered the non-resistance training, it is time to move on to resistance training, in which you squeeze your PFM against the opposing force of resistance in an effort to accelerate the PFMT.

If you are challenged by the non-resistance PFMT or cannot or prefer not to use resistance—which requires the placement of a device in your vagina—you can continue with the non-resistance training using it as a "maintenance" program. PFM maintenance training requires continuing with the PFMT program, but performing it less frequently, twice weekly usually being sufficient.

PFMT Programs

What follows are the programs that I have designed based on my specialized training and medical experience, and influenced by interactions with physical therapists, exercise experts, Pilates and yoga instructors and most importantly my patients. Programs have been crafted to treat areas of PFM weakness, e.g., if strength is the issue, emphasis on strength training is in order, whereas if PFM stamina is the issue, focus on endurance training is appropriate.

There are few, if any, programs in existence that are designed for specific pelvic floor dysfunctions, so I have created "tailored" PFMT exercise routines, customized for the particular pelvic health issue at hand, including SUI, OAB, POP, sexual/orgasm issues and pelvic pain.

These programs are *not* designed with the intent that they be rigidly adhered to as they can be customized to make them work for *you*, recognizing that every woman and every pelvic floor is unique. You can modify the programs and experiment with all variables—intensity, power, contraction and relaxation duration, number of reps and number of sets, with the ultimate objective of challenging the PFM to make them stronger, better toned, firmer and healthier.

Do what feels right and works for you, building to your maximum potential over time. If you feel fatigued before completing the number of reps recommended, do as many quality contractions as you can do. If you cannot maintain contraction intensity for the duration recommended, do the best you can. Three sets per session are ideal, but if you find this too challenging, you can do two sets or even just one. If you find that completing 3 sets becomes a simple task, you can do 4 or 5 sets as your PFM become stronger and more durable.

There are three basic types of PFM contractions based upon the duration and intensity of the contraction. Three "S" words make these contractions easy to remember: **Snaps, Shorts** and **Sustained.**

Snaps are rapid, high intensity pulses of the PFM that take less than one second per cycle of contracting and relaxing. These are the type of PFM contractions that occur involuntarily at the time of sexual climax, so should be easy to understand and perform.

Shorts are slower, less intense squeezes of the PFM that can last anywhere from two to five seconds (with equal time allotted to the relaxing phase).

Sustained PFM contractions are less intense squeezes that last ten seconds or longer (with an equal time in the relaxing phase). These are the type of PFM contractions that you use when you have a strong desire to urinate or move your bowels but do not have access to a bathroom and must apply effort to "hold it in."

Before starting the PFMT program, I recommend a warm-up week to practice and become familiar with snaps, shorts and sustained contractions. Do not start the formal PFMT until you feel comfortable with all three contractions. Do the Oxford strength and endurance testing to obtain baseline values before you begin the warm-up week (See Chapter 12 to review the details of the testing).

If your Oxford grade is 0-2, consider yourself to have weak PFM. If you cannot do more than 20 snaps, 15 shorts or one-10 second sustained contraction, consider your endurance poor. If your PFM strength is good, but your endurance is poor, use the program tailored for poor endurance. If you have a specific pelvic dysfunction that you would like to focus on improving, use the program tailored to that specific dysfunction. If you suffer with more than one pelvic floor dysfunction, e.g., both POP and SUI, determine which issue is most compelling and disturbing to you and start with that specific program. If you feel that the problems are equal in degree, complete one program followed in succession by the other.

Warm-Up Week: Do as many good quality snaps as possible until you feel that you can no longer do them with full intensity. Take a short break and then do as many good quality shorts until you feel that your efforts are diminishing. Finally, do a sustained contraction for as long as you can until fatigue sets in. After a short break, repeat the sustained contraction. Do this warm-up every other day for this preliminary week before proceeding with the programs.

General PFMT Program

*The general program is a balanced program that incorporates strength and endurance training. It is intended for women who are found to have poor PFM strength or poor strength and endurance on the preliminary testing. It is also appropriate for women **without** specific pelvic issues who wish to pursue a PFM exercise program to make their PFM stronger, more durable and to help prevent the onset of pelvic floor issues.*

Perform the following: 3 sets; one-minute break between each set; do 3-4 times weekly; with each week try to step up the intensity of the PFM contractions and duration of the short contractions; allot equal time to relaxing phase as contracting phase; refer back to previous pages if you need a refresher on snaps, shorts and sustained.

Week 1: snaps x20; 2-5 second shorts x15; 10 second sustained x1 = 1 set

Week 2: snaps x30; 2-5 second shorts x20; 10 second sustained x2 = 1 set

Week 3: snaps x40; 2-5 second shorts x25; 10 second sustained x3 = 1 set

Week 4: snaps x50; 2-5 second shorts x30; 10 second sustained x3 = 1 set

Week 5 and on: Advance to resistance training (see following chapter).

However, if you were severely challenged by this non-resistance program or cannot or prefer not to use resistance—which requires the placement of a device in your vagina—you can continue this as a "maintenance" program, consisting of the Week 4 regimen performed twice weekly (as opposed to every other day).

PFMT for Poor PFM Endurance

This program is designed for those with satisfactory PFM strength (Oxford grades 3-5), but poor endurance. The number of contractions performed and contraction duration are gradually increased over the course of the training program as adaptation occurs.

Perform the following: 3 sets; one-minute break between each set; do 3-4 times weekly; allot equal time to relaxing phase as contracting phase.

Week 1: snaps x15; 2 second shorts x15; 6 second sustained x1 = 1 set

Week 2: snaps x25; 3 second shorts x20; 8 second sustained x2 = 1 set

Week 3: snaps x35; 4 second shorts x25; 10 second sustained x3 = 1 set

Week 4: snaps x50; 5 second shorts x30; 10 second sustained x4 = 1 set

Week 5 and on: Advance to resistance training (see following chapter).

If you found yourself severely challenged by this non-resistance program or cannot/prefer not to use resistance (which requires the placement of a device in your vagina), you can continue this as a "maintenance" program consisting of the Week 4 regimen performed twice weekly (as opposed to every other day).

PFMT for POP/Vaginal Laxity

Endurance training is especially relevant for those with POP and poor vaginal tone. Focusing on sustained contractions will benefit the slow twitch endurance PFM fibers that are the prime contributors to pelvic tone and support.

Perform the following: 3 sets; one-minute break between each set; do 3-4 times weekly; with each successive week, work on stepping up the intensity of the PFM contractions; allot equal time to relaxing phase as contracting phase.

Week 1: snaps x20; 2-5 second shorts x15; 10 second sustained x1 = 1 set

Week 2: snaps x30; 2-5 second shorts x20; 10 second sustained x2 = 1 set

Week 3: snaps x40; 2-5 second shorts x25; 10 second sustained x3 = 1 set

Week 4: snaps x50; 2-5 second shorts x30; 10 second sustained x4 = 1 set

Week 5 and on: Advance to resistance training (see following chapter).

However, if you were severely challenged by this non-resistance program or cannot or prefer not to use resistance—which requires the placement of a device in your vagina—you can continue using this as a "maintenance" program, which will consist of the Week 4 regimen performed twice weekly (as opposed to every other day).

PFMT for Sexual/Orgasm Issues

The PFM contract intensively at the time of climax with each contraction lasting about 0.8 of a second, about how long a snap lasts. A series of vigorous snaps is precisely the PFM contraction pattern experienced at the time of orgasm. If you have issues with achieving an orgasm or with orgasm intensity, this natural contraction pattern is replicated in this program, which focuses on high-intensity pulses of the PFM (snaps) that benefit the fast twitch explosive fibers. Endurance training is also important for sexual function since sustained contractions benefit the slow twitch endurance PFM fibers that contribute to pelvic support and vaginal tone.

Perform the following: 3 sets; one-minute break between each set; do 3-4 times weekly; with each week work on stepping up the intensity of the snap PFM contractions; allot equal time to relaxing phase as contracting phase.

Week 1: snaps x30; 2-5 second shorts x15; 10 second sustained x1 = 1 set

Week 2: snaps x40; 2-5 second shorts x20; 10 second sustained x2 = 1 set

Week 3: snaps x50; 2-5 second shorts x25; 10 second sustained x3 = 1 set

Week 4: snaps x60; 2-5 second shorts x30; 10 second sustained x4 = 1 set

Week 5 and on: Advance to resistance training (see following chapter).

However, if you were severely challenged by this non-resistance program or cannot/prefer not to use resistance—which requires the placement of a device in your vagina—you can continue using this as a "maintenance" program, consisting of the Week 4 regimen performed twice weekly (as opposed to every other day).

PFMT for SUI

Strength and power training are critical for managing SUI, with the power element (i.e., how rapidly you can maximally contract your PFM) vital in order to react quickly to SUI triggers. Focusing on moderate intensity contractions that last for several seconds (shorts) will benefit SUI, as this type of PFM contraction deployed prior to and during any activity that induces the SUI will help prevent its occurrence. Attention directed to these short contractions will allow earlier activation of the PFM with SUI triggers, as well as increased contraction strength and durability to counteract the sudden increase in abdominal pressure that induces SUI. Effort applied to sustained contractions is equally important since the slow twitch endurance PFM fibers are prime contributors to pelvic tone and pelvic support of the urethra, which promote urinary continence.

Perform the following: 3 sets; one-minute break between each set; do 3-4 times weekly; with each successive week try to step up the PFM contraction intensity as well as the activation speed (how long it takes to get to peak intensity); allot equal time to relaxing phase as contracting phase.

Week 1: snaps x20; 5 second shorts x15; 10 second sustained x1 = 1 set

Week 2: snaps x30; 5 second shorts x20; 10 second sustained x2 = 1 set

Week 3: snaps x40; 5 second shorts x25; 10 second sustained x3 = 1 set

Week 4: snaps x50; 5 second shorts x30; 10 second sustained x4 = 1 set

Week 5 and on: Advance to resistance training (see following chapter).

However, if you were severely challenged by this non-resistance program or cannot or prefer not to use resistance—which requires the placement of a device in your vagina—you can continue this as a "maintenance" program, which consists of the Week 4 regimen performed twice weekly (as opposed to every other day).

PFMT for OAB and Urinary/Bowel Incontinence

Focusing on high-intensity pulses of the PFM (snaps) will benefit the fast twitch explosive fibers that are critical for inhibiting urinary and bowel urgency/urgency incontinence. These snaps will generate increased PFM strength and power to enhance the inhibitory reflex between PFM and the bladder/bowel, permitting a speedy reaction to urgency and facilitating the means to counteract urinary and bowel urgency, frequency and incontinence. Of equal importance is endurance training of the slow twitch, fatigue-resistant fibers that contribute to baseline tone of the voluntary urinary and bowel sphincters.

Perform the following: 3 sets; one-minute break between each set; do 3-4 times weekly; with each successive week try to step up the intensity of the PFM contractions; allot equal time to relaxing phase as contracting phase.

Week 1: snaps x20; 2-5 second shorts x15; 10 second sustained x1 = 1 set

Week 2: snaps x30; 2-5 second shorts x20; 10 second sustained x2 = 1 set

Week 3: snaps x40; 2-5 second shorts x25; 10 second sustained x3 = 1 set

Week 4: snaps x50; 2-5 second shorts x30; 10 second sustained x4 = 1 set

Week 5 and on: Advance to resistance training (see following chapter).

However, if you were severely challenged by this non-resistance program or cannot/prefer not to use resistance (which requires the placement of a device in your vagina), you can continue using this as a "maintenance" program, which will consist of the Week 4 regimen performed twice weekly (as opposed to every other day).

PFMT for Pelvic Pain Due to Tension Myalgia: "Reverse" PFMT

Focusing on the relaxing aspect of the PFM contraction/relaxation cycle is the key to "down-train" the PFM from their over-tensioned, knot-like state. Those with over-contracted and over-toned PFM will not benefit from the typical strengthening PFMT done for most PFM dysfunctions—and can actually worsen their condition—so the emphasis here is on the relaxation phase of the PFM. This is "reverse" PFMT, conscious unclenching of the PFM in which the PFM drop and slacken as opposed to rise and contract. Reverse PFMT strives to stretch, relax, lengthen and increase the flexibility of the PFM.

"Reverse" Kegels can be a confusing and difficult concept, particularly because these exercises demand conscious relaxation of the PFM, which only occurs subconsciously in real life. Recall that the PFM have a baseline level of tone and that complete PFM relaxation only occurs at the time of urination, bowel movements, passing gas or childbirth.

To make this easier to understand, think of a PFM contraction on a scale of 0-10, with 0 being complete relaxation and 10 being maximal contraction. I have arbitrarily chosen 2 as the baseline level of PFM tone. In reverse Kegel exercises you strive to go from 2 to 0 as opposed to standard exercises in which the effort is to go from 2 to 10. When you urinate, move your bowels or pass gas, the PFM relax to a level of 0, so this is the feeling that you should strive to replicate, while continuing to breathe regularly without straining or pushing. A deep exhalation of air will facilitate PFM relaxation, as it does for other muscle groups.

Perform the following: A very gentle PFM contraction to initiate PFM engagement, followed by deep relaxation and release of the PFM lasting as long as the contraction; 3 sets; one-minute break between each set; do 3-4 times weekly.

Week 1: reverse snaps x20; reverse 2-5 shorts x15; reverse 10 second sustained x1 = 1 set

Week 2: reverse snaps x30; reverse 2-5 shorts x20; reverse 10 second sustained x2 = 1 set

Week 3: reverse snaps x40; reverse 2-5 shorts x25; reverse 10 second sustained x3 = 1 set

> **Week 4: reverse snaps x50; reverse 2-5 shorts x30; reverse 10 second sustained x3 = 1 set**

Week 5 and on: There is no role for using resistance exercises for tension myalgia. Continue using this program as a "maintenance" program, consisting of the Week 4 regimen done twice weekly (as opposed to every other day). Make a concerted effort at keeping the PFM relaxed at all times, not just while pursuing the PFMT program.

Integrating PFMT Into Other Exercise Routines

Initially, it is important to isolate the PFM and exercise them while not actively contracting any other muscle groups. Once PFM mastery is achieved, PFM exercises can then be integrated into other exercise routines, workouts and daily activities. In real life, muscles do not work in isolation, but rather as part of a team. The PFM are no exception, often contracting in conjunction with the other core muscles in a mutually supportive way, co-activating to maintain lumbar-pelvic stability, help prevent back pain and contribute to pelvic tone and strength. Core training that exercises the abdominal/lumbar/pelvic muscles as a unit improves the PFM response. Many Pilates and yoga exercises involve consciously contracting the PFM together with other core muscles during exercise routines.

Dynamic exercises in which complex body movements are coupled with core and PFM engagement provide optimal support and "lift" of the PFM, enhance non-core as well as core strength and heighten the mind-body connection. When walking, gently contract your PFM to engage them in the supportive role for which they were designed, which will also contribute to good posture. Contract the PFM when standing up, climbing steps, doing squats and lunges, marching, skipping, jumping, jogging, dancing and cycling.

The core muscles—including the PFM—stabilize the trunk when the limbs are active, enabling powerful limb movements. It is impossible to use arm and leg muscles effectively in any athletic endeavor without engaging a solid core as a "platform" from which to push off. Normally this happens without conscious effort; however, with focus and engagement, the core and PFM involvement can be optimized. The stronger the core platform, the more powerful the potential push off that platform will be, resulting in more forceful arm and leg movements. Thus, maximizing PFM strength has the benefit of optimizing limb power.

Weight training and other forms of high impact exercise can result in tremendous increases in abdominal pressure. This force is largely exerted downwards towards the pelvic floor, particularly when exercising in the standing position, when gravity comes into play, potentially harmful to the integrity of the PFM. Engaging the PFM during such efforts will help counteract the downward forces exerted on the pelvic floor. "Compensatory" PFM contractions, in which the PFM are contracted in proportion to the increased abdominal pressure, are effective in balancing out the forces exerted upon the pelvic floor.

Putting Your PFMT Into Action

Functional pelvic fitness is the practical and actionable means of applying PFM proficiency to common everyday activities in order to improve pelvic function. It encompasses the knowledge of how to contract and relax PFM muscles through their full range of motion in the real world (as opposed to isolated, out-of-context contractions), when to do so, how much to do so and why to do so. For many women, this is the essence of PFMT--having stronger and more durable PFM to improve their quality of life. These purposeful and consciously applied PFM contractions are not intended as exercise or training—although they will secondarily serve that purpose—but as management of the various pelvic floor dysfunctions at the times and moments that the problems become apparent. When practiced diligently, these targeted PFM contractions can ultimately become automatic (reflex behaviors).

When you feel the sudden and urgent desire to urinate or move your bowels, snap your PFM several times, briefly but intensely. When your PFM are so engaged, the bladder muscle reflexively relaxes and the feeling of intense urgency should disappear. Understand that this is most effective when the bladder or bowels are not full, but are contracting involuntarily.

For urgency incontinence, prior to trigger exposure—hand washing, key in the door, arising from sitting, running water, entering the shower, cold or rainy weather, etc.—snap your PFM rapidly several times to preempt the involuntary bladder contraction before it occurs (or diminish or abort the bladder contraction after it begins).

With respect to SUI, by actively contracting the PFM immediately before exposure to the activity that prompts the SUI, the incontinence can be improved or prevented. For example, if changing position from sitting to standing results in SUI, do a brisk few-second duration PFM contraction prior to and when transitioning from sitting to standing to brace the PFM and pinch the urethra shut.

If you have POP and have defined activities that cause the prolapsed pelvic organ to drop or protrude—often standing, bending or straining—engage the PFM prior to or during these triggers. If you need to manually reduce the POP (by pushing the prolapse in with your fingers), after doing so, consciously engage the PFM to maintain the prolapsed pelvic organ in its proper anatomical position.

Integrate your newfound PFM powers in the bedroom and intensify your sensation as well as his by gradually tightening your vaginal "grip" around his penis during sexual intercourse. Alternatively, you can pulse your PFM rhythmically while pelvic thrusting or pulse your PFM without pelvic thrusting, the snapping providing penile stimulation in the absence of active thrusting. As you develop increasing PFM proficiency, you may be able to selectively contract individual PFM in isolation, simultaneously, or in such a sequence that can result in a titillating experience for both you and your partner. You may be able to develop as much fine motor control of your vagina as you have for your fingers and hands! At the time of sexual climax, focus on the involuntary rhythmic contractions of your PFM and try to heighten the experience by explosively contracting them.

If you suffer with tension myalgia of the PFM, focus on consciously unclenching the PFM over the course of your day. Be particularly aware of the natural PFM relaxation that occurs when urinating or moving your bowels and strive to replicate that feeling of PFM release.

14 PFM RESISTANCE TRAINING

"In the preservation or restoration of muscular function, nothing is more fundamental than the frequent repetition of correctly guided exercises instituted by the patient's own efforts. Exercise must be carried out against progressively increasing resistance, since muscles increase in strength in direct proportion to the demands placed upon them."

—JV Luck
Air Surgeon's Bulletin, 1945

"Resistance exercise is one of the most efficient ways to stimulate muscular and metabolic adaptation."

—Mark Peterson, PhD

Resistance

Resistance training is a means of strength conditioning in which work is performed against an *opposing force*. The premise of resistance training is that by gradually and progressively overloading the muscles working against the resistance, they will adapt by becoming bigger and stronger. PFMT using resistance optimizes PFM conditioning, resulting in more power, stability and endurance and the functional benefits to pelvic health that accrue. It also helps to rebuild as well as maintain PFM mass that tends to decrease with aging.

Applying Resistance Training to the PFM

Resistance is easy to understand with respect to external muscles, e.g., it is applied to the biceps muscles when you do arm curls with dumbbells. Resistance training can be applied to the PFM by contracting your PFM against a compressible device placed in your vagina. Its presence gives you a physical and tangible object to squeeze against, as opposed to basic training, which exercises the PFM without resistance. Resistance PFMT is similar to weight training—in both instances, the adaptive process gradually but progressively increases the capacity to do more reps with greater PFM contractility and less difficulty completing the regimen. In time, the resistance can be dialed up, accelerating the adaptive process.

Recall that in the late 1940s, Dr. Arnold Kegel devised the *perineometer* that enabled resistance PFM exercises. It consisted of a pneumatic vaginal chamber connected by tubing to a pressure manometer. This device provided both a means of resistance and visual biofeedback. The chamber was inserted into the vagina and the PFM were contracted while observing the pressure gauge (calibrated from 0-100 mm mercury). With training, the PFM strength increased in proportion to the measured PFM contractions.

PFMT Resistance Tools

There are many PFM resistance devices on the market and my intention is to provide information about what is available, but NOT to endorse any product in particular. What follows is by no means a comprehensive review of all products. Some are basic and simple, but many of the newer ones are "high tech" and sophisticated means of providing resistance, biofeedback and tracking, often via Bluetooth connectivity to a smartphone. I classify the devices into vaginal weights, electro-stimulation devices, simple resistance devices and sophisticated resistance devices. Within each category, the devices are listed in order of increasing cost.

Vaginal Weights

These weighted objects are placed in the vagina and require PFM engagement in order that they stay in position. They are not intended to be used with any formal training program, but do provide resistance to contract down upon.

Vaginal Cones: This consists of a set of cones of identical shape but variable weights. Initially, you place a light cone in your vagina and stand and walk about, allowing gravity to come into play. PFM contractions are required to prevent the cone from falling out. The intent is to retain the weighted cone for fifteen minutes twice daily to improve the strength of the PFM. Gradual progression to heavier cones challenges the PFM. (Search "vaginal cones" as there are several products on the market.)

WHO KNEW?   *Be careful not to wear open-toed shoes when walking around with the weighted cones ... a broken toe is a possible complication!*

Ben Wa Balls: These are similar to vaginal cones, but appear more like erotic toys than medical devices. There are numerous variations on the theme of weighted balls that can be inserted in your vagina, available in a variety of different sizes and weights. Some are attached to a string, allowing you to tug on the balls to add more resistance. Another type has a compressible elastic covering that can be squeezed down upon with PFM contractions. Still others vibrate. There are some upscale varieties that are carved into egg shapes from minerals such as jade and obsidian. (Search "Ben Wa Balls.")

WHO KNEW?   *Vaginal Kung Fu. Kim Anami is a life and sex coach who advocates vaginal "weightlifting" to help women physically and emotionally "reconnect" to their vaginas and become more in tune with their sexual energy. Her weightlifting has included coconuts, statues, conch shells, etc. According to her, vaginal weightlifting increases libido, lubrication, orgasm potential and sexual pleasure for both partners.*

Electro-Stimulation Devices

These devices work by passive electrical stimulation of the PFM. Electrical impulses trigger PFM contractions without the necessity for active engagement.

WHO KNEW?   *Many clinical studies have shown that electro-stimulation in conjunction with PFMT offers no real advantages over PFMT alone. Like the electrical abdominal belts that claim to tone and shape your abdominal muscles with no actual work on your part, these devices seem much better in theory than in actual performance.*

Intensity: This is a battery-powered erotic device that looks like the popular "rabbit" vibrator sex toy. It consists of an inflatable vaginal probe that has an external handle. It has contact points on the probe that electro-stimulate the PFM and vibrators for both clitoral and "G-spot" stimulation. It has 5 speeds and 10 levels of stimulation. Cost is $199 (Pourmoi.com).

ApexM: This device is intended for use by patients with SUI. It consists of an inflatable vaginal probe and control handle. You insert it inside your vagina, inflate it for a snug fit and power it on. Electric current is used to induce PFM contractions. The intensity is increased until a PFM contraction occurs, after which the device is used 5-10 minutes daily. Cost is $299 (Incontrolmedical.com).

Simple PFMT Resistance Devices

These are basic model, inexpensive resistance devices. They consist of varying physical elements that you place in your vagina to give you a tangible object to contract your PFM upon. They provide biofeedback to ensure that you are contracting the proper muscles. Some offer progressive resistance while others only a single resistance level.

These devices can be used in conjunction with the specific programs that were specified in Chapter 13. To do so, repeat the 4-week program for your specific pelvic floor dysfunction while incorporating these devices into the regimen. You may discover that the 4-week programs using the devices that offer progressive resistance become too challenging as you dial up the resistance level. If this is the case, you can continue with the first week's program while increasing the resistance over time. Customize and modify the programs to make them work for you, as was recommended for the tailored programs without using resistance.

Educator Pelvic Floor Exercise Indicator: This is a tampon-shaped device that you insert into your vagina. It is attached to an external arm that moves when you are contracting the PFM properly, giving you positive feedback. Cost is $32.99 on Amazon (Neenpelvichealth.com).

Gyneflex: This is a flexible V-shaped plastic device that is available in different resistances. You insert it in your vagina (apex of the V first) and when you squeeze your PFM properly, the external handles on each limb of the V close down, the goal being to get them to touch. Cost is $39.95 (Gyneflex.com).

WHO KNEW? *The Gyneflex is similar in form and function to hand grippers that increase grip strength.*

Pelvic Toner: Manufactured in the UK, this is a spring-based resistance device that you insert into your vagina. It has an external handle and two internal arms that remain separated, so the device must be held closed and inserted. When your hold is released the device springs open and, by contracting your PFM, you can close the device. It offers five different levels of resistance. Cost is 29.99 British pounds (Pelvictoner.co.uk).

Magic Banana: This is a PFM exerciser that consists of a loop of plastic and silicone tubing joined on a handle end. The loop is inserted in the vagina and squeezed against. When the PFM are contracted properly, the two arms of the loop squeeze together. Cost is $49.99 (Magicbanana.com).

KegelMaster: This is a spring-loaded device that you insert in your vagina and is squeezed upon. It has an external handle with a knob that can be tightened or loosened to provide resistance by clamping down or separating the two arms of the internal component. Four springs offer different levels of resistance. Cost is $98.95 (Kegelmaster.com).

WHO KNEW? **WHAT? "Kegel Pelvic Muscle Thigh Exerciser": This is a Y-shaped plastic device that fits between your inner thighs. When you squeeze your thighs together, the gadget squeezes closed. This exerciser has NOTHING to do with the PFM as it strengthens the adductor muscles of the thigh, serving only to reinforce doing the wrong exercise and it is shameful that the manufacturer mentions the terms "Kegel" and "pelvic muscle" in the description of this product.**

Sophisticated PFMT Resistance Devices

These are complex and often expensive devices that provide resistance, biofeedback and tracking, often via Bluetooth connectivity to a smartphone. Many provide specific PFMT programs to follow for optimal results.

Lovelife Krush: Made by sex technology company OhMiBod, this is a dumbbell-shaped device that you insert vaginally and connect via Bluetooth to a companion app TASL (The Art and Science of Love). Its voice-guided training program tracks PFM contraction pressure, endurance and number of reps and provides vibrational stimulation as you perform the exercises. Cost is $129 (Lovelifetoys.com/lovelife-krush).

kGoal: Its name is a play on the word "Kegel." It is an interactive "smart" device that consists of an inflatable and squeezable plastic "pillow" that is attached to an external handle. It provides feedback, resistance and tracking. You insert the pillow in your vagina and inflate or deflate it with a button control to obtain a good fit. When you contract your PFM properly, the device vibrates to give you biofeedback. The kGoal app can be downloaded on your smartphone and connected to the device via Bluetooth. The interface provides a guided workout including pulses, 5-second holds and slow and deliberate holds. It provides visual and auditory feedback and tracks your progress. The device measures the strength of your vaginal contractions and at the end of a workout you receive a score of 1-10 to help monitor your progress. Cost is $149 (Minnalife.com).

Vibrance Kegel Device: This biofeedback tool can be set at different resistance levels and provides audio guidance and coaching. It consists of a pressure-sensitive element that you insert in your vagina. When you contract your PFM properly, it delivers mild vibrational pulsations. It has three different training sheaths of increasing stiffness that provide graduated levels of resistance for different training intensities. Cost is $165 (VibrancePelvicTrainer.com).

Elvie: Manufactured in the UK, Elvie is a wearable, egg-shaped, waterproof, flexible device that you insert in your vagina. Your PFM contraction strength is measured and sent via Bluetooth to a companion mobile app that provides biofeedback to track progress. Five-minute workouts are designed to lift and tone the PFM. The app includes a game designed to keep users engaged by bouncing a ball above a line by clenching their PFM. The carrying case also serves as a charging device. Cost is $199 (Elvie.com).

PeriCoach: Manufactured in Australia, PeriCoach is a vaginal device that measures PFM contraction strength, which is relayed to your smartphone via Bluetooth to a companion mobile app. It provides a guided exercise program, data monitoring and audio-visual biofeedback. It is available only by prescription. Cost is $299 (PeriCoach.com).

InTone: This device must be prescribed by a physician and is specifically for SUI and OAB. It combines voice-guided PFM exercises with visual biofeedback and electro-stimulation. It consists of an inflatable vaginal probe that provides resistance and measures PFM contractile strength. The probe is attached to a handle and a separate control unit furnishes the guided program and biofeedback. An illuminated bar graph displays the strength of your PFM contractions and objective data to track your progress. Exercise sessions are 12 minutes in length. Cost is $795 (Incontrolmedical.com).

WHO KNEW? *As reported in the International Journal of Urogynecology, a 3-month clinical trial of the InTone device resulted in significant subjective and objective improvements in patients with SUI and OAB.*

Do I really need to use a resistance device?

You can strengthen your PFM and improve/prevent pelvic floor dysfunction without using resistance, so it is not imperative to use a device that is placed in the vagina in order to derive benefits from PFMT. Some women are unwilling or cannot place a device in the vagina. However, since muscle strengthening occurs in direct proportion to the demands placed upon the muscle, using resistance is the most efficient means of accelerating the adaptive process, as recognized and espoused by Dr. Kegel. There is a real advantage to be derived from squeezing against a compressible device as opposed to against air. Furthermore, the biofeedback that many of the resistance devices provide is invaluable in ensuring that you are contracting your PFM properly and in tracking your progress.

Which resistance device will work best for me?

There are many resistance devices available in a rapidly changing, competitive and evolving market. Most of the sophisticated training devices provide the same basic functionality—insertion into the vagina, connection to a smartphone app, and biofeedback and tracking—although each device has its own special features. The goal is to find a device that is comfortable and easy to use. Some devices are more medically-oriented whereas others are more sex toy-oriented. Each has unique bells and whistles, some offering programs with guidance and coaching and a few incorporating games to make the PFMT process entertaining. I urge you to visit the website of any device that you might be interested in to obtain more information. Read their reviews in order to make an informed choice as to which product is most appropriate for you.

15 CONCLUDING WORDS: NEW PARADIGM

People whose diseases are prevented as opposed to cured may never really appreciate what has been done for them. Zimmerman's law: Nobody notices when things go right.

—Walter M. Bortz II, M.D.
Next Medicine: The Science and Civics of Health

Achieving a fit pelvic floor by strengthening and toning the PFM—the "hidden jewels" of the pelvis—is a first line approach that can improve a variety of pelvic maladies in a way that is natural, accessible and free from harmful side effects. Although it is advantageous to treat the symptoms of pelvic floor dysfunction, it is another dimension entirely to take a proactive approach by strengthening the PFM in an effort to prevent pelvic floor dysfunction.

Pregnancy, labor, childbirth, aging, menopause, weight gain, gravity, straining and chronic increases in abdominal pressure take their toll on pelvic anatomy and function, affecting vaginal tone, support of the pelvic organs, urinary and bowel control and sexual function. Although humans have a remarkable capacity for self-repair and pelvic issues can be dealt with after the fact, why be reactive instead of being proactive? Why not attend to future problems before they actually become problems? Isn't a better approach "an ounce of prevention is worth a pound of cure"? Why not pursue a strategy to prevent pelvic floor dysfunction instead of fixing it, not allowing function to become dysfunction?

In the USA, over 350,000 surgical procedures are performed annually to treat two of the most common pelvic floor dysfunctions—SUI and POP. Estimates are that by the year 2050, this number will rise to more than 600,000. These sobering statistics provide the incentive for changing the current treatment paradigm to a preventive pelvic health paradigm with the goal of avoiding, delaying or diminishing deteriorations in pelvic floor function.

If birth trauma to the pelvic floor often brings on pelvic floor dysfunction as well as urinary, bowel, gynecological and sexual consequences, why not start PFMT well before pregnancy? This runs counter to both our repair-based medical culture that is not preventive-oriented and our patient population that often opts for fixing things as opposed to preventing them from occurring.

Realistically, PFMT prior to pregnancy will not prevent pelvic floor dysfunction in everyone. Unquestionably, obstetrical trauma (9 months of pregnancy, labor and vaginal delivery of a baby that is about half the size of a Butterball turkey, repeated several times) can and will often cause pelvic floor dysfunction, whether the PFM are fit or not! However, even if PFMT does not prevent all forms of pelvic floor dysfunction, it will certainly impact it in a very positive way, lessening the degree of the dysfunction and accelerating the healing process. Furthermore, mastering PFM exercises before pregnancy will make carrying the pregnancy easier and will facilitate labor and delivery and the effortless resumption of the exercises in the post-partum period, as the exercises were learned under ideal circumstances, prior to PFM injury. Since there are other risk factors for PFM dysfunction aside from obstetric considerations, this preventive model is equally applicable to women who are not pregnant or never wish to become pregnant.

Preventive health paradigms are commonly practiced with respect to general physical fitness. We work out not only to achieve better fitness, but also to maintain fitness and prevent losses in strength, flexibility, endurance, balance, etc. In this spirit, I encourage those of you who are enjoying excellent pelvic health to maintain this health with a preventive PFMT program. For those readers working to improve your pelvic health, continue forward on the journey. Regardless of whether your goal is treatment or prevention, a PFMT program will allow you to honor your pelvic floor and become empowered from within.